EXTRAORDINARY CENTENARIANS IN AMERICA

Their secrets to living a long vibrant life

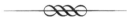

GWEN WEISS-NUMEROFF

Agio
PUBLISHING HOUSE

Agio
PUBLISHING HOUSE 151 Howe Street,
Victoria BC Canada V8V 4K5

*For rights information and bulk
orders, please contact* us through
agiopublishing.com

Extraordinary Centenarians in America
is based on the recollections of the people
commemorated in this book as well as
their closest family members. Due to the
possibility of human error, the author
cannot guarantee the complete accuracy
of the information. It should also be noted
that since the time the interviews were
conducted, some of these individuals have
passed away. The author expresses her
condolences to their loved ones and hopes
this book will serve as a reminder of their
incredible legacy.

Although nutrition and lifestyle data has
been collected and reported, the author is
not dispensing medical advice or calling
this a scientific study. The intent of the
author is to provide information for
readers to consider in consultation with
their health practitioners.

Visit Gwen Weiss-Numeroff's website at
www.livingvibrantlyto100.com

A portion of the
author's royalties
will be donated
to the Ovarian Cancer
Research Fund.

Extraordinary Centenarians in America
ISBN 978-1-897435-86-1 (paperback)
ISBN 978-1-897435-87-8 (hardcover)
ISBN 978-1-897435-88-5 (ebook)

Cataloguing information available from
Library and Archives Canada.
Printed on acid-free paper.
Agio Publishing House is a socially
responsible company, measuring success
on a triple-bottom-line basis.
10 9 8 7 6 5 4 3 2 1a

DEDICATION

In memory of my beloved mother and brother. Your spirits guided me throughout.

THE CENTENARIAN PHENOMENON

According to the most recent Census data, there are currently almost 62,000 people who have reached the age of 100 living in the United States. There are five times as many centenarian women than there are men. In fact, centenarians are now the second fastest growing demographic segment in the country, second only to the super-centenarians (those at least 110 years of age).

While much attention has been given to the number of centenarians living in Japan, the United States has more centenarians than any other country in the world. Upper-nonagenarians, or those living between 95 and 99, are increasing rapidly as well, up over 30% versus a decade ago. There are over 398,000 American upper-nonagenarians.

Longevity itself is one of the greatest advances of the 20th century, with the average life span nearly 30 years longer compared to the century prior. Now, with even greater medical advances, the promise shown by new stem cell research, recent genetic breakthroughs and many new initiatives solely focused on centenarians, an even greater increase in longevity is certainly possible.

According to the Gerontology Research Group and *Guinness Book of World Records*, the oldest verified person that ever lived was Jeanne Calment from France, who died at 122 years and 164 days old. At the time this book was written, there were only four Americans among the top 100 oldest people that ever lived. You will get to know two of these Americans in the following pages: Besse Cooper, 116, the world's oldest living person and Dr. Leila Denmark, 114, the world's fourth oldest.

Let's look through a small window at what life was like in the United States of America when our centenarians were born versus today:

YEAR	1912	2012
US Population	92 million	312 million
Life Expectancy	Male 48.4 years, Female 51.8	Male 75.7, Female 80.6
Average Salary	$750/year	exact number unknown but significantly higher
National Debt	$1.15 billion	$16+ trillion
Divorce	1 out of 1000	1 out of 2
Vacation	12-day cruise $60	$600+
Milk	$.32/gallon	$3.20+

Sources: Lone Star College-Kingwood Library – kclibrary.lonestar.edu; 2011 Census Bureau; Centers for Disease Control and Prevention; *Guiness Book of World Records*; divorce statistics from Jennifer Baker; Forest Institute of Professional Psychology, Springfield; Bureau of Labor Statistics; usgovernmentdebt.us

ACKNOWLEDGEMENTS

It took 2 years of searching to find this extraordinary group of individuals from all walks of life who fit a certain criteria—lived in America for at least 75 years, 100 years old (give or take a few years), lived healthily most of their lives and vibrantly into their 90s, 100 and beyond.

Thank you to all of those remarkable individuals for generously sharing your lives with me, from your childhood memories to your nutritional habits. You were all such honest, accessible and truly lovely people. Thank you for your captivating stories and words of wisdom. They will remain in my mind and in my heart always and will certainly inspire countless others.

I would also like to thank those who led me to some of these incredible people, whether it was by sending me media clippings, personal referrals or actual introductions—you all are greatly appreciated: Irving Ladimer and Bel Kaufman (both profiled in this book), Stacey Cusick, Dr. Moises Fraifeld, Diane Greenspan, Ro Miller, Nicole Futterman, David Weiss, Betty Turner, Debra Harten and Alisa Destefano.

Special thanks to my wonderful husband, Bruce, who was always on the lookout for extraordinary centenarians, willingly accompanied me on some of my longer trips and supported me throughout the entire process. My partner and best friend for life, may we be together as long and as strong as the inspiring people in this book.

— *Gwen Weiss-Numeroff*

I would like to introduce you to an extraordinary group of Americans. Their ages range from 96 to 116. Each is exceptional in unique ways and they all share one thing in common – an infectious spirit and the ability to inspire. These individuals will truly help diminish your fear of aging, as they not only have lived long, they have lived vibrantly.

Please refer to the *Reaching 100 and Beyond!* tables at the end of each chapter for information on each subject's family history and lifestyle factors. This information was provided by the subjects themselves and some of their family members.

TABLE OF CONTENTS

Introduction   i

Featured Centenarians:

GARDNER WATTS
Teacher, Tennis Player, Museum Founder   2

BEL KAUFMAN
Novelist, Teacher, Granddaughter Of Sholem Aleichem   8

BESSE COOPER
Teacher, The Oldest Person In The World   16

ANTHONY MANCINELLI
World's Oldest Barber   22

RUTH GRUBER
Photojournalist, Author, Humanitarian, Heroine   28

DR. LEILA DENMARK
Pediatrician, Co-Developer Of The Whooping Cough Vaccine   36

BONITA ZIGRANG
Professional Singer, Dental Assistant, Matriarch   44

BENJAMIN GOLDFADEN
Former NBA Player, Teacher, Insurance Salesman   50

SAMUEL 'ERRIE' BALL
Pro Golfer, Sole Survivor of 1st Masters Tournament   58

ALYSE LAEMMLE
Life Insurance Agent   64

IRVING KAHN
The World's Oldest Active Investment Professional   74

HELEN MULLIGAN
Factory Worker   82

EBBY HALLIDAY
Real Estate Legend   88

GILBERT HERRICK
WWII Veteran, Postal Worker, Eternal Bachelor (almost)   98

Lillian Modell & Gussie Levine   104

GUSSIE LEVINE
Teacher, Author of Children's Books   106

LILLIAN MODELL
Bookkeeper, Secretary, "Working Girl"   110

JENNIE CASCONE
Seamstress   116

MURRAY H. SHUSTERMAN
Attorney, Philanthropist   122

ANNE LOMEDICO
Book Binder, Adventurer   130

ANNE LAMONT
Dancer   136

MORRIS LENSKY
Traveling Salesman, Family Man   142

A Bronx Tale:
A Celebration of Their Hometown Centenarians   148

IRVING LADIMER
Attorney, Professor, Civic Leader   152

JOHANNA ZURNDORFER
Survivor, Caregiver, Advocate For The Needy   158

LORETTA HODGE
Nanny, Housekeeper (For Bette Davis And Patrick O'Neal) 164

OSCAR CHAIKIN
Salesman, Business Owner, Caulbearer   172

HILDA SCHWALL BERNER
Secretary, Community Leader   180

MIRIAM HENSON
Homemaker, Caretaker, Retail Clerk   186

BARBARA BRODY
Singer, Actress, Artist, Teacher   194

WINIFRED THOMAS
Nanny, Housekeeper, Minister   200

SANDRA HOROWITZ
School Secretary, WAC Soldier   206

How have they lived so long, and so well?   214

About the author   227

INTRODUCTION

My intense fear of illness and loss started when I was 8, when the closest person in the world to me, my big brother Steven, died of leukemia. He was 9. During the four years of his illness, everyone in our family knew that he was dying except for me, and Steven. The family did not have the emotional strength to tell us. I was completely devastated and it changed my life's path forever.

While I was in my 20s, my dear Uncle Jerry died at 48 of a heart attack; he also had multiple sclerosis. His daughter, my cousin Janice, died a few years later of a bad case of asthma; she was 28. Then the grandparents died, three of them were in their 60s and early 70s, although one managed to live to 79 years old, and she was the sickest of them all.

Moving into my 30s and early 40s, my best friend and maid of honor, Tammy, died of breast cancer at 33. My friend and devoted secretary for 6 years, Jean, died of a blood disease in her early 50s. Then Uncle Herbie died in his 60s, and Aunt Irma in her early 70s, both from disease.

The final straw was when I was 45, three years ago. My mother fell ill from ovarian cancer at 70. Doctors diagnosed it just 3 weeks before she died. The sudden loss left me devastated once again.

I needed some answers and, more importantly, some hope!

The fear of illness and losing loved ones had been looming over my head since that fateful day at 8 years old. I had been studying nutrition since my teens trying to find ways to prevent such a devastating loss from happening again. I also studied psychology to see if there were emotional factors that contributed to disease and decreased longevity. Most studies indicated that there was indeed a significant correlation between diet, stress, mental attitude and disease.

Over the next decades I began to walk the talk. I ate a healthy, balanced diet and became very active in tennis and yoga, significantly decreasing my stress level. I began taking life more in stride, truly appreciating my blessings, and in the midst of all this, the looming fear began to diminish and I started to feel a sense of control over my health and joy in my life.

I began my career in advertising due to my interest in consumer behavior, but not surprisingly ended up in the health and wellness field. I founded a corporate wellness company to teach large groups of working individuals how to reach their optimal health and balance. I started working with schools, lecturing to children about increasing their energy through quality food, and advised administrations about improving the school food. Eventually, I started my own private practice, coaching individuals to live a healthy, vibrant life.

This path was working. I was helping people improve their health, productivity and well-being and my own physical and emotional health was better than I could ever have imagined, particularly given my family history.

However, questions about longevity still lingered in my mind. It was my mother's abrupt death that incited me to actively search out people who were living examples of my ultimate dream for my family, my clients and for myself. I needed to meet those who have lived a long, healthy and vital life. I wanted to meet people in my own country, not in Okinawa, Japan, or some other remote region where the culture, water or diet were so different from my own. I wanted to hear their incredible stories of what they had witnessed in their lives, how they dealt with so much loss witnessed simply because of their longevity. I wanted to hear their words of wisdom given their vast life experience and, most importantly, learn *"How they got to be so old?"*

Unlike today, people in their generation regularly died from polio, influenza, diabetes, asthma, high blood pressure—if they survived childbirth! The average life expectancy of those born before the first world war was only 50. These individuals have exceeded all expectations, doubling the norm—how did they do it?

Was it just genetic, did their lifestyle have anything to do with it, or their personalities? What were the commonalities, if any, amongst them? And what on Earth could they possibly be doing to pass their time at such an old age?

I poured through various news and social media, and asked hundreds of people for anyone they knew who fit my criteria: 100 years old, give or take a few years, still generally healthy and mentally engaged.

As I started locating these extreme elders, what I found was truly amazing! I found centenarians, upper-nonagenarians (96-99) and even some super-centenarians (110+) in this country who were not only still healthy and alert, they had been living strong, vibrant lives in their 80s, their 90s and even into their 100s! Still working, driving, volunteering, traveling, writing, doing things they had never done before in their lives, in their "platinum"* years! After hearing about some of these folks, my criteria shifted. I was no longer just looking for healthy and mentally engaged centenarians, I was now searching for vibrant, *extraordinary* centenarians.

As I grew to know this amazing group of people and many of their family members, who generously welcomed me into their lives, I was beyond inspired. Each one of these people was outstanding in a unique way.

In their presence, I felt my old fear of illness and aging quickly melting down, and I felt hopeful! I learned that I just might not be doomed by my genetics after all, and that there is so much more to do and accomplish in the coming decades of my life. I will cherish their incredible stories, wonderful personalities, and words of wisdom, even the quirky ones, for the rest of my life.

* *'Platinum' is defined in this book as those years 80 and beyond.*

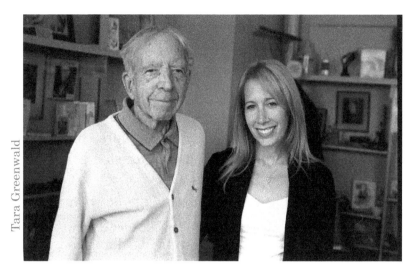

Gardner Watts and the author at the Suffern Village Museum founded by Watts and his wife, Josephine.

My first interviewee was Mr. Gardner Watts. I discovered him in our local (Rockland County, New York) newspaper as he had recently climbed the Statue of Liberty, by stairs—from the base to her crown. He was 96 years old at the time.

My hope is that these extraordinary Americans will not only fascinate you, but help diminish your fear of aging, inspire you to think more positively about your future, furnish you with ideas of what you can do in the latter chapters of your life, and motivate you to take better care of your mind, body and spirit.

Reaching 100 doesn't necessarily mean physical or mental disability, nor does it mean, in some cases, retirement. These people are helping to redefine aging in new and inspirational ways.

EXTRAORDINARY
CENTENARIANS
IN AMERICA

Teacher, Tennis Player, Museum Founder
Born: April 3, 1914, in Patterson, New York
Current residence: Suffern, New York

GARDNER WATTS

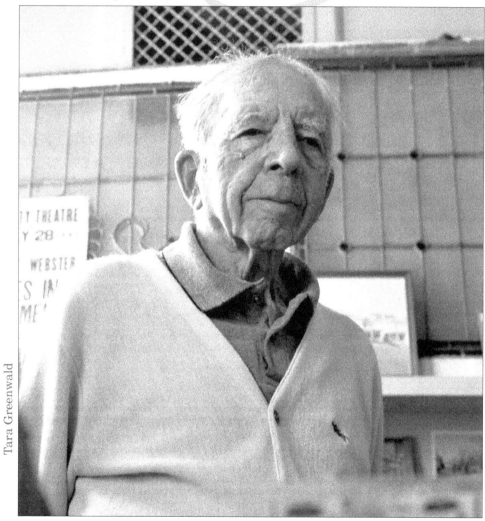

Tara Greenwald

Words of Wisdom

98

"My longevity is attributed to my long, happy marriage. We did everything together. She was perfect in my eyes."

In my search to find extraordinary centenarians, I scoured the Internet, newspapers, network and cable television, social networks, my own networks, you name it. I was looking for not only those that have lived for a century, but those that are still living it up! On the way, I heard about a few upper nonagenarians (those in their late 90s) who were so incredible, I decided that they were close enough to the century mark to still inspire and amaze my readers.

I found my first prospective subject, Gardner Watts, in our local newspaper and he was the epitome of whom I was searching for. Gardner was in the media not because he was celebrating a monumental birthday; he was featured because he had just climbed the Statue of Liberty by stairs at 96 years old! Yes, Gardner climbed 354 stairs, 270 feet, and was singled out by three National Park

Rangers as being the oldest person to climb from ground level to the base of her crown with no use of the elevator. (Access to the crown had just been reopened after an eight-year closure following the Sept 11, 2001, terror attacks just across the New York harbor.)

Bright, well-rounded and talented

Gardner is regarded as somewhat of a celebrity in the Rockland County area. He was a World War II veteran and a local high school history teacher for 36 years, founded and led the Historical Hikers for 50 years, was tennis coach at the high school for 25 years and was 4-time Rockland County Tennis Doubles champion. Gardner was also the winner of a Fulbright Scholarship for his academic merit which enabled him to live and teach in Finland with his wife and 5 children for one year.

A love story like no other

After winning several scholarships, Gardner attended Amherst College and then Columbia for his master's degree in history. After a one-year stint teaching in impoverished Puerto Rico where "many of my youngsters came to school barefoot," Gardner had the opportunity to teach in his hometown where he soon met his wife, Josephine. Gardner met her at the library and took her "to a square dance and skiing" on their first date. They soon fell in love and got married, but just weeks after their nuptials in 1942, Gardner was drafted into the US Army. Incredibly, in order to be closer to her beloved husband, Josephine enlisted in the Army as well, and due to her strong

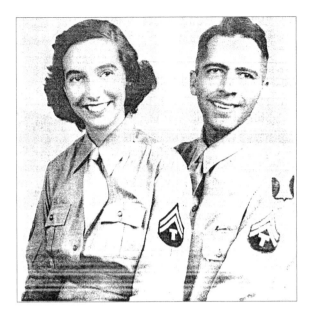

Gardner during his military years with his wife, Josephine. Photo courtesy of Gardner Watts

academic background was soon assigned to breaking secret Japanese codes outside of Washington, DC.

When I visited with him at the Suffern Village Museum, which he and his wife founded, Gardner spoke so passionately about his beloved Josephine, it was as if they were newlyweds. He adamantly believes that his close, loving marriage contributed to his longevity. As we walked around the museum, he led me to a female mannequin clothed in a US Army uniform with a dog tag (metal military identification tag) around its neck; both were Josephine's. Josephine passed away at 86 years old in 2006. They were married 64 years.

Overcoming life's challenges

Gardner was in college during the Great Depression. "In my hometown, the effect of the Depression was profound. At 50, after spending his entire career as a minister, my father lost his pastorate because the church could no longer afford to pay his salary. There was a great deal of unemployment here; it was a very serious time." Fortunately, Gardner's academic career was protected due to his many scholarships.

Gardner also witnessed the Ku Klux Klan frequently marching outside of his father's church.

In the US Army, Gardner was stationed in Panama. On the way to reach his posting, "we were attacked by Nazi U-boats and spent

At age 70, Gardner and his wife founded the Suffern Village Museum with a team of residents and he still oversees the museum.

two days with our life jackets on waiting for more Nazi attacks."

As with all of our centenarians profiled in this book, Gardner has had his share of loss; his parents, his wife, one of his children, his sibling and, of course, many friends. However, his wonderful attitude and zest for life enabled him to continue on to do extraordinary things.

Golden years activities

After retiring, the last thing Gardner did was sit around. At age 70, Gardner and his wife founded the Suffern Village Museum with a team of residents and he still oversees the museum and its many treasured pieces. In his late 90s, Gardner is still active and adventurous. He took up kayaking a few years ago with his daughter and has for years enjoyed canoeing with his friends. Up until a few years ago, he was still avidly playing tennis and recently went hot air ballooning with a female friend. Gardner most recently was selected as one of the Top 100 Scouters (Boy Scouters) in Hudson Valley.

His father was the founder of the Boy Scouts in his town and trained with one of the national founders of the Boy Scouts of America, Dan Beard. Gardner feels that being involved with the scouts has helped define him as a man. "When I was a boy, your life was your school, the church and scouting."

Lastly, as we all know, Gardner still hikes, his most recent, up to the crown of the Statue of Liberty.

At the end of our interview and photo session, I happened to ask Gardner if he ever used a cane. He proudly replied, "Never, just a hiking stick."

Lifestyle

General Health	Gardner always led a clean, active life and had a positive mental attitude. His general health was excellent.
Smoking	Never.
Alcohol	Never.
Nutrition	Gardner's mother and wife always made home-cooked wholesome meals. He ate a "variety of foods, no big portions, no overeating, ate lots of hot cereal, eggs, nothing extreme either way."
Physical activity	Gardner was always active and still is. He was an avid tennis player and still hikes, canoes and kayaks. He was never overweight.
Current interests	Gardner still drives, plays pool, loves to read and plays piano. He often goes to the library and sees friends. The weekend of this interview, Gardner was going to a Halloween party with a friend dressed as an explorer (very apropos).
Family	Gardner is very close with his remaining 4 children, 8 grandchildren, 2 great grandchildren, and 86-year-old brother.

Family History

	AGE OF DEATH	CAUSE OF DEATH
Mother	84	car accident
Father	63	intestinal cancer
Brother	53	unknown
Brother	n/a	living, age 86

Novelist, Teacher, Granddaughter Of Sholem Aleichem

Born: May 10, 1911, in Berlin, Germany

Current residence: Manhattan, New York

BEL KAUFMAN

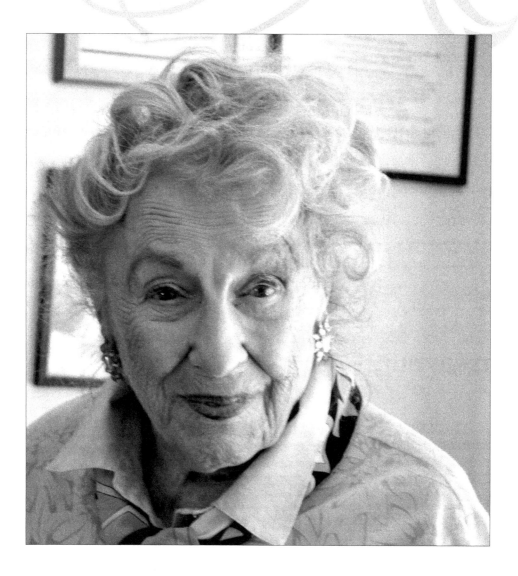

101
Words of Wisdom

"Laughter keeps you healthy. You can survive by seeing the humor in everything. Thumb your nose at sadness; turn the tables on tragedy. You can't laugh and be angry, you can't laugh and feel sad, you can't laugh and feel envious. And there is always something funny, if you have the eyes to see it."

Bel Kaufman was gifted. Her grandfather, Solomon Naumovich Rabinovich, was a famous author and playwright, known by his pen name Sholem Aleichem (it means "peace be with you"). Sholem Aleichem's stories inspired the marvelous musical *Fiddler on the Roof*. It was apparent after meeting with Bel that she indeed inherited her grandfather's genes of humor and creativity, traits which came in handy throughout her life.

Whether it was growing up during the Russian Revolution or struggling as a teacher in the inner city schools, Bel always found a way to look past the difficulties and see the humor in it all. This talent was central to her tremendous success as the author of the novel *Up the Down Staircase*, based loosely on her life as a teacher in New York City. Her novel sat on the *New York Times* Best Seller

> *"I frequently would come upon dead bodies in the street frozen in grotesque postures. Didn't every child do that?"*

list for well over a year and was adapted to both film and stage. The book was set during early racial integration and busing, and dealt with the difficulties of bureaucracy, student indifference and teacher incompetence, yet was told in a humorous way that resonated with readers all over the country.

The success of this book led to her second career as a lecturer, just like her grandfather, in venues filled with people who wish to hear her words of wisdom about surviving darkness with laughter.

Here is how her story unfolds…

The Russian Revolution though the eyes of a child

Bel was born in Germany where her father was studying medicine. When she was just a young girl, the family moved to Odessa in Russia during the heat of the Russian Revolution. There, she said, she would "frequently come upon dead bodies in the street, frozen in grotesque postures." She explained, "A child has no basis for comparison: Didn't every child do that? I took it for granted that that's how children lived." Young Bel also saw nothing unusual about standing in line for a ration of *green* bread. "There was no flour, so the bread was made from the shells of peas."

"In Odessa," she recalls, "every other week there was a new government—Bolshevik, Stalinist, Leninist. During the communist Bolshevik regime, I was wheeling my little brother in his carriage in front of my house and two young communist women in leather jackets approached me. They proceeded to take my brother out of the carriage, plopped him into my 9-year-old skinny arms, took the carriage, and said to me (in Russian), 'We also have babies!' I went crying to my mother with my brother in my arms. She asked me what happened, and I replied, 'They have babies, too!'

"Militia would enter homes, break things, take things. We decided

10

to leave Russia, not because we were Jews, but because we were something worse to them—bourgeois. My father was a doctor; we had a house, a cook. Many of my father's colleagues were jailed, even killed."

In 1923, at age 12, Bel and her family managed to flee Russia, thanks partly to the enduring prestige of her grandfather, Sholem Aleichem, who had died 7 years earlier. Even through wars and revolutions, Sholem Aleichem had been incredibly famous. He was a renowned Yiddish writer who spun the bittersweet Tevye stories that later became the source for *Fiddler on the Roof*. He was so beloved in Russia, the US and Israel that his face appeared on postage stamps and coins, streets in Russia and Israel were named after him, many monuments of him were erected, and more than 100,000 people attended his funeral, more than any other in New York City history, where he died. When Bel's mother pleaded with the authorities to allow

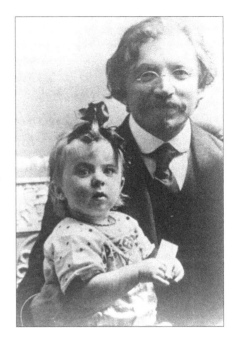

Young Bel and her grandfather, Sholem Aleichem. Photo courtesy of Ms. Kaufman

"I watched unemployed men selling pencils and apples on the street."

her to visit her mother, Aleichem's widow, who was living in the US, not surprisingly, they obliged.

Moving to the USA

When Bel and her parents moved to the United States, they dealt with the challenges of learning a foreign language and boarding with unfamiliar relatives in a strange new place. As soon as she graduated high school, amidst the Great Depression, she fled straight to Manhattan on her own. "When I first moved here," she recalled, "I paid only $4.50 a week for rent and ate at Automats. I watched unemployed men selling pencils and apples on the street."

She has lived in New York City ever since.

A relentless woman

Bel learned enough English to graduate from Hunter College, magna cum laude, and received her master's degree from Columbia University with high honors. She was offered various PhD programs, but had fallen in love with a medical student (who eventually became her first husband), and turned her back on academia to work and support him through school. The work she had chosen was teaching.

"From then on, they (the Board of Ed) only assigned poems from dead poets."

You need a license to teach in New York City public schools. Despite the degrees and honors Bel had achieved, the Board of Education kept failing her on the oral examination because of her strong Russian accent. She attended a year of speech classes and, finally rid her accent, passed the oral.

Despite this achievement, the Board of Ed rejected her again because they didn't like her interpretation of the assigned test poem. Not one to back down, she mustered her chutzpah and contacted the poet herself. The long letter she got back included the poet's warm praise of her interpretation, which she sent along to the Board of Ed. Thoroughly chastened, the Board finally gave Bel her license to teach. Bel notes, "From then on, they only assigned poems from dead poets."

An accidental best seller

While she was struggling to get her teaching license, Bel wasn't idle. She spent years as a "permanent sub" (substitute) working in some of the city's worst schools. The experience provided the material—literally—for her future best-selling novel *Up the Down Staircase*. She found her best ideas going through classroom wastebaskets gathering notes the students had written on scraps of paper. Although the subject of her book was serious, she wrote it with humor and affection, a gift inherited from her famous grandfather.

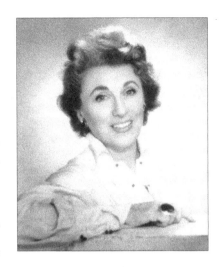

Author Bel in her earlier years. Photo courtesy of Ms. Kaufman

Her novel later became a play and a movie, and was translated into 16 languages.

A woman by any other name...

Bel was the first female writer whose work was published in *Esquire* magazine. She employed a bit of subterfuge to achieve that honor: she chopped off the last two letters of her name, Belle, hoping that the publishers would assume "Bel" was a man's name. It turned out to be unnecessary; even when they found out, they liked her short stories so much they published them anyway. The new version of her name became her byline for the rest of her life.

Still so much to do

At 101, Bel is still writing short stories, some about her grandfather, and lectures widely, passing along what she has learned about surviving through humor. She's been interviewed on the *Today* show, featured in a documentary, *Laughter in the Darkness*, about her grandfather's life, and a documentary is currently in the works about her own life.

> "I'll never retire [from working] as long as I live—that's like retiring from life!"

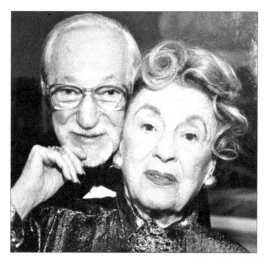

Bel and her "husband," Sidney Gluck. Photo courtesy of Ms. Kaufman

She is adamant on the subject of retirement: "I'll never retire as long as I live—that's like retiring from life! I'll never stop writing, teaching, lecturing. If you're in good health, living is exciting on its own."

Bel shares a Manhattan apartment with her second "husband," Sidney Gluck, 95, whom she never technically married. Bel and Sidney have been together for 40 years since her divorce. What is the secret to their long, loving relationship? "We don't do anything together. His interests are so different from mine. He is an authority on China, lectures about the country, and has a TV program about it. He also runs the Sholem Aleichem foundation." She adds playfully, "He also likes older women."

A year before he died in 1916, Sholem Alechiem wrote to Bel: "Dear Babushka, I'm writing you this letter to ask you to hurry up and grow so that you can write me a letter. In order to do this, you must drink milk, eat vegetables and soup, and fewer candies." At 101, she still intends to answer his letter.

> Bel loves reaching 100. "For the first time in my life, I don't have to do what someone else says I have to do. If I don't recognize people, I have an excuse—I just say I'm 100 years old!"

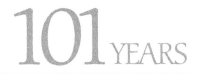

Lifestyle

General health	Bel has never had a serious illness in her life. Even when her appendix was taken out, it was found to be healthy. (Her father, a doctor, kept it in a jar.)
Smoking	Smoked three packs a day for 40 years, finally quitting at age 60.
Alcohol	An occasional social drink.
Nutrition	Bel's diet is better now, but "I was brought up during famine, so I have enormous respect and love for food. I ate everything, including junk food. But I didn't overeat, and I weigh today the same as when I was 20." She takes 2,000 mg of vitamin C on a regular basis.
Physical activity	Bel has always loved dancing, and still does ballroom dancing for 90 minutes every week. When she was young she stayed fit by climbing poles.
Current interests	Bel writes funny poems and short stories; "doodles"; reads avidly; lectures to teachers, Jewish groups and writers; and, until recently, traveled all over the world.
Family	Bel has one daughter and one son. They don't live nearby but she speaks with them on a regular basis. She has one granddaughter and sees her brother regularly, who lives a few blocks away. He calls her every morning to start her day off with a funny joke.

Family history

	AGE OF DEATH	CAUSE OF DEATH
Mother	76	bladder cancer
Father	67	stroke
Brother	n/a	living, age 91

Teacher, The Oldest Person In The World

Born: August 26, 1896, in Sullivan County, Tennessee

Current residence: Monroe, Georgia

BESSE COOPER

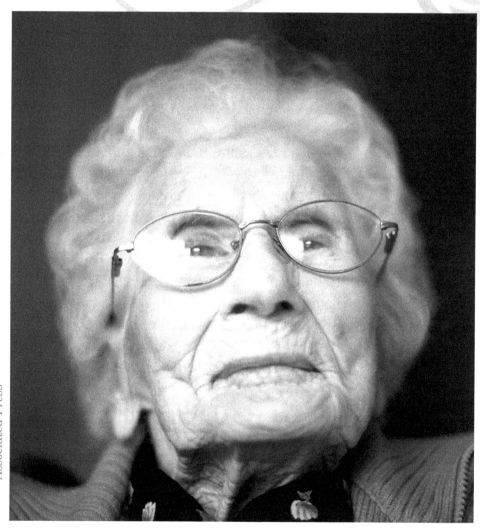

Associated Press

116 Words of Wisdom

"Mind your own business and don't eat junk food. Treat everyone the way you want to be treated, work hard and love what you do."

Besse Cooper is a super-centenarian (over 110 years of age). Her memory has diminished to some extent, so this interview was conducted and information garnered with the assistance of Besse's son, Sidney Cooper, who is presently 76.

The Oldest Person in the World

On June 21, 2011, following the death of Brazilian super-centenarian Maria Gomes Valentim, Besse Cooper of Monroe, Georgia, took the coveted role of becoming the world's oldest living person. Six months later, after Japanese super-centenarian Chiyono Hasegawa died, she also became the last living person born in 1896. Besse is one of only 24 people who has ever lived past 115 years.

Going Outside of the Box

Besse grew up on a farm in a small community outside of Gotham City, Tennessee. In 1916, she was one of the first people to attend East Tennessee State Normal School. During that period of time in the South, "normal schools" were quite popular. They were essentially two-year schools started primarily to train teachers. There she received her teaching degree, one of the proudest moments of her life. Her son Sydney recalls, "In those days, it was unheard of for a lady who lived eight miles outside of the city to go to college. Mom was a country girl but had an aunt who lived in the city. She would live with her aunt and come home on the weekends via train. Back then you typically rode a boat, buggy or wagon, never a train."

> "There was no electricity so there was no utility bill to worry about. We just had to purchase kerosene for the lamps, a little salt, sugar and pepper. Everything else, we raised."

Besse taught in Tennessee for three years, but at 22, she decided to move to Georgia as they paid teachers a higher salary. Ten years later, when her first child was born, she decided to stay home to raise her children, four in total. Besse was married to Luther Cooper for nearly 40 years until his death at only 68 years old. She never remarried.

Learned to do without

The most difficult time for Besse was living through the Great Depression. They learned to do without, but they were more fortunate as they lived on a farm and produced all of their own food. According to Sidney, "There was no electricity so there was no utility bill to worry about. We just had to purchase kerosene for the lamps, a

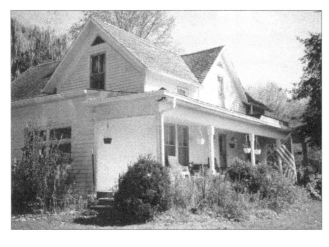

Besse's family house built in 1906 in Boones Creek, TN. Photo courtesy of Besse Cooper

little salt, sugar and pepper. Everything else, we raised. We didn't have electricity until 1946 as they had stopped building lines for electricity due to the war."

A wholesome country girl

When Besse moved to Georgia, she preferred to stay true to her roots. Hence, she and Luther purchased a house surrounded by 50 acres of farmland. It cost them $500. Besse rigorously tended to the farm every day. She ate off of the farm for nearly every meal, eating fresh, organic meats, fruits, vegetables and bread. And, unlike most of her siblings whose lives were cut short from heart disease and cancer, Besse never smoked or consumed alcohol a day in her life.

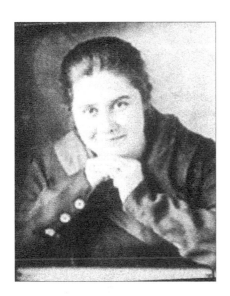

Besse in her earlier years. Photo courtesy of Besse Cooper

Following her husband's death, Besse continued to reside at their beloved farm until she was 105.

Always active and mentally engaged

Well into her centenarian years, Besse still tended to her large flower and vegetable garden, read avidly, kept up with politics and loved solving crossword puzzles. She loved to cook and, according to Sidney, "she would make the best apple jelly you ever ate in your life." In her 80s, she became involved with the local senior center and traveled extensively with her daughter, primarily for free, as her daughter worked for Delta Airlines. They travelled the country visiting various relatives in different states. She still says, "the 80s were the best years of my life!"

At 105, she moved to an assisted living center and in January of 2003, at 107, conceded to accept full-time assistance and moved into a nursing home. At 116 years old, she has lost some of her vision and hearing, but all of her vital signs are still good. Says Sidney, "She amazes the doctors and nurses. She still gets up for breakfast and lunch, and always gets dressed for dinner, but is now in bed most of the time."

Sidney adds, "Mother was always a very strong person due to her father's influence. He would say, 'If you set your mind to do something, you could do it.' Mother was never a worrier or complainer and was always positive."

REACHING 100 & BEYOND!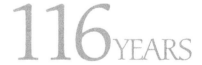

Lifestyle

General health	Was in good health her entire life and, at 116, her vital signs are still good.
Smoking	Never.
Alcohol	Never.
Nutrition	Consumed all kinds of pasture-raised meat, eggs, fresh produce which they froze and ate all year long. All foods were eaten moderately. Had no desire for junk food, just fresh, low-fat popcorn. Oatmeal most mornings and never deep-fried anything. Rarely ate out.

Physical activity	Worked outdoors on the farm every day.
Current interests	Until 18 months ago when she lost some of her vision and hearing, she watched the news every night, kept up with politics, read avidly (especially the Bible) and loved to work on crossword puzzles. She tended to her flower and vegetable garden until she was 102.
Family	Besse's son, Sidney, visits her a few times a week, and one of her grandsons visits her five days per week. Sidney says, "My son is completely fascinated with her and I think the stimulation from him has contributed to her longevity." Her 12 grandchildren, 15 great and one great-great visit her as well.

Family history

	AGE OF DEATH	CAUSE OF DEATH
Mother	62	heart failure
Father	72	unknown
Sister	88	kidney cancer
Brother	75	heart attack
Sister	70s	stomach cancer
Brother	early 70s	throat cancer
Brother	68	lung cancer
Brother	23	heart defect
Sister	4	unknown

Note of interest: one of Besse's grandfathers died in the Civil War.

World's Oldest Barber

Born: March 2, 1911, in Monte Melone, Italy

Current residence: New Windsor, New York

ANTHONY MANCINELLI

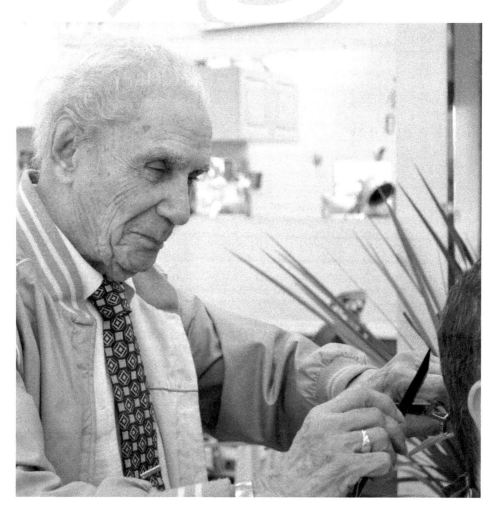

Anthony Mancinelli still cutting hair at age 101.

101 Words of Wisdom

"Do the right thing, don't smoke, don't drink, eat right and don't overdo it. If you need a little extra help, take some vitamins. Going to work is what keeps me going."

A ntonio and Pasquale Mugnano, the refreshingly passionate, heavily-accented Italian-American owners of the barbershop bearing their names, proudly introduced me to their most famous employee.

Employee of the century

This is the man who holds the title from the *Guinness Book of World Records* as the world's oldest working barber. Anthony Mancinelli is a tall, very lean man with a full head of white hair. He also possesses one of the warmest smiles I have ever encountered. I immediately was comfortable in his presence and felt as if I was meeting a man decades younger. At age 101, Anthony still lives independently, drives himself to work every week and does not require eyeglasses.

"My dad wasn't making much money and had seven kids to feed. I wanted to help out so I gave my parents all of my earnings, except for my tips, which I saved for presents for them. I gave them $5 to $7 per week."

He is extraordinarily sharp and alert for a man of any age and attributes this to "chatting with thousands of people for 88 years as a barber."

A barber at 12 years old

Anthony was born on a farm right outside of Naples, Italy and lived with his grandfather, who lived to be 103. Granddad didn't die from natural causes. He was climbing a ladder to pick figs from a tree and died from injuries after falling. Says Anthony, "Before he died, my grandfather said to me, 'If you live to be 103, don't climb a tree!'"

Anthony's family moved to the US when he was 9 years old. He enjoyed being around barbershops and started learning the trade from the local barbers when he was just 12. He would wake up at 4:30 a.m. to deliver the morning papers, eat breakfast, go to school, deliver afternoon newspapers, and then went off to the barber shop to learn the business until 8 p.m. He then went home, ate dinner and went to bed as, "I had to get up at 4:30 all over again."

The reason he worked so hard as a child? "My dad wasn't making much money and had seven kids to feed. I wanted to help out so I gave my parents all of my earnings, except my tips, which I saved for presents for them. I gave them $5 to $7 per week by making 3 cents per paper. I started cleaning the barber shop at

"I just like to come in and meet the customers. Going to work is what keeps me going."

first and made a couple of dollars per week there as well."

"However, everything was cheap then, milk was 5 cents, bread 6 cents, a haircut and shave 25 cents (or 2 bits). I finally gave up on the papers and stayed with the barber business and have been working ever since. I like to meet different people."

Anthony owned his first barbershop when he was 20 years old. After 6 years, he moved to a different location where he stayed for about 50 years. When local gangs began to loiter around his shop, he sold it and started working for other barbershops in the surrounding area until he settled at Antonio & Pasquale's where he is still snipping away.

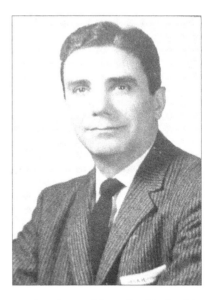

Anthony Mancinelli in his early years. Photo courtesy of Mr. Mancinelli

"I've cut the hair of young boys, their father's hair, their grandfather's hair and sometimes even their great-grandfather's hair." Customers say he is like a walking history book—with stories of the Great Depression, WWII and several Yankee championships. Some customers have sat in his chair literally hundreds of times.

There was a short break in his barbershop tenure in 1945 when Anthony served in the Army near the end of World War II. He was stationed in the US for one year inspecting the troops before they went overseas to see if they had everything they needed. He married his longtime love, Carmela, and was wed for 69 years. She passed away 6 years ago at the age of 89. Anthony had two sons, one of whom tragically died at 43 of an aneurysm.

Still chatting with customers after 88 years

Anthony is not planning on retiring and sitting all day in front of a television. He charges $12 for a haircut and some regular customers have said his fingers are still just as nimble. He works typically one day a week now, but would like to work every day. "I just like to come in and meet the customers, going to work is what keeps me going."

Anthony describes himself as easy-going, someone who "goes with the tide." At 101, Anthony is still very independent. He cooks for himself, cleans his own apartment, mends his own clothes, does his own laundry and is on no medication. He has an excellent memory: "I remember all of the principals in every school," has perfect hearing and keen vision. In fact, he even cuts his own hair.

REACHING 100 & BEYOND! 101 YEARS

Lifestyle

General health	Anthony is on no medication, has an excellent memory and still has good hearing and vision.
Smoking	Never.
Alcohol	Only on a special occasion.
Nutrition	Eats moderately and has never been overweight. He enjoys plenty of greens, particularly dandelion greens, pasta, soups, his own marinara sauce, meat (on occasion) and his own lasagna. He drinks no soda, but enjoys green tea. He has also been taking multivitamins for about 40 years.
Physical activity	Nothing regimented, but always moving, busy, cutting hair, standing.

Current interests	Cutting hair, used to garden frequently, still likes to cook.
Family	Anthony had two sons, one died at 43 of an aneurysm and his other son is currently 74 years old. He has 6 grandchildren and 6 great-grandchildren who he sees regularly.

Family history

	AGE OF DEATH	CAUSE OF DEATH
Mother	71	blood disease
Father	81	heart attack
Brother	n/a	living, age 89
Sister	89	natural causes
Brother	79	diabetes
Brother	70s	unknown sickness
Brother	60	hunting accident
Brother	27	unknown sickness
Son	43	aneurysm

"Anthony possesses one of the warmest smiles I have ever encountered."

Photojournalist, Author, Humanitarian, Heroine
Born: September 30, 1911, in Brooklyn, New York
Current residence: Manhattan, New York

RUTH GRUBER

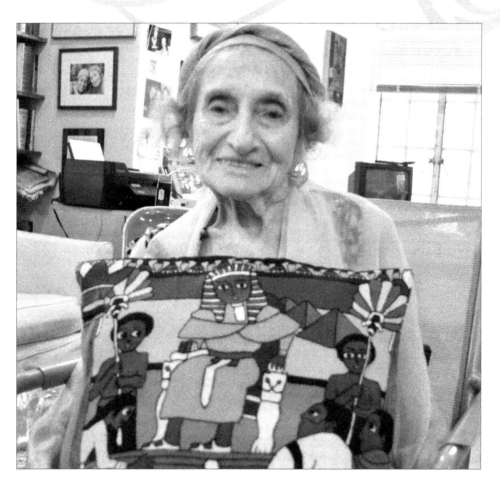

Ruth Gruber holding a pillow handcrafted by one of the many
Ethiopian Jews she helped save from persecution.

Words of Wisdom

101

"Look inside your soul and find your tools. We all have tools and have to live with the help of them. I have two tools, my words and my images. I used my typewriter, computer and my cameras to fight injustice. Whenever I see a possibility of helping people who are in danger, I want to help them."

As I entered Ms. Ruth Gruber's lovely, expansive apartment overlooking Central Park, I was surrounded by a colorful collection of artwork and mementos, book-lined shelves and a poster of a recently-released movie based on her extraordinary life.

A true humanitarian

There were numerous awards for her writing and humanitarian efforts. Included was the Golda Meir Human Rights Award, National Jewish Book Award for Best Book on Israel, National Coalition against Censorship Award for her work defending free expression, Distinguished Journalist Awards and so on.

What also caught my attention was her beautiful collection

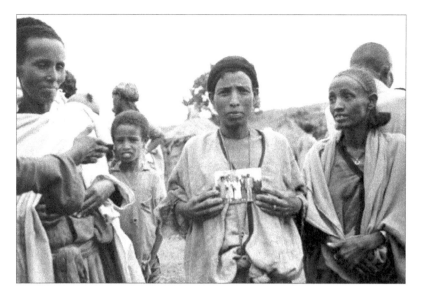

Ruth Gruber's photo of Ethiopian Jews during the Big Exodus in the 1980s. Photo courtesy of Ms. Gruber

of pillows and throws made of boldly-colored fabrics with African scenes on them. When I asked Ruth about them, she proudly informed me that they were handmade by Ethiopian Jews as they were waiting to flee Ethiopia. In 1985, while in her 70s, Ruth was involved in a mission to free these Jews from poverty and persecution and to relocate them to Israel. Ruth and others taught them how to craft these items to sell and help pay for their education and other expenses.

Ruth has devoted most of her life to helping those in need, and those who have been persecuted and needed assistance fleeing their own countries. She used her talents of writing and photography as her "tools" to accomplish these goals.

"It is amazing how one teacher can change your entire life."

Ruth is a tiny woman, not quite 5 feet tall with a warm smile and an air of someone wise, gracious and patient with my questioning. She had a quiet, soft presence, her voice just a whisper, a stark contrast to the tough, resilient woman in her earlier years.

A strong academic presence starts in first grade

Ruth spoke very highly of her family and how successful her siblings had become. When I asked if there was anyone who had inspired her family to succeed, she responded, "In our family, the top of the totem pole was the rabbi, then the teacher, then your parents." She paused, then added, "When I was in first grade, my teacher came to my house. My mother asked what I did wrong. The teacher said to my mother, 'Take good care of her, she is going to be a writer.' That was in 1st grade when we were taught poetry by this teacher. Most teachers did not do that. From then on, I just fell in love with poetry, reading and writing. It is amazing how one teacher can change your life." And what a changed life it was.

"My mother was convinced she would never see me again."

Ruth went to college at New York University (at $3 a credit for tuition) and then received her Masters degree in Wisconsin. "I hitchhiked from Brooklyn to Wisconsin. My father allowed me to as it was for my education—everyone hitchhiked in those days."

After receiving her Masters degree, she applied for a fellowship to study in Germany. She had taken German as her first language in college simply because she loved Bach and Beethoven.

In 1931, at 19, Ruth received a fellowship from The Institute of International Education. "My family was opposed to me going to Germany as it was already clear in America that Hitler was doing damage. My mother was convinced she would never see me again."

However, Ruth had the scholarship funds and was determined to go. "My mother thought Hitler would come down and shoot me, so I said I would carry my American flag in my lapel and my American passport in my brassiere. 'Hitler can't shoot me through a passport!' I told her."

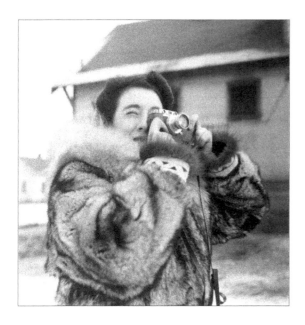

Ruth Gruber in her early years as a photojournalist. This photo was used to promote the recent documentary about her life, Ahead of Time. *Photo courtesy Ruth Gruber*

In spite of the rising anti-Semitism in Germany, Ruth went there and became the youngest person in the world ever to receive her doctorate, a PhD, at age 20.

She states emphatically, "Since then, my mantra became, 'never let obstacles stop you'."

Triumphing over challenges

Called "a 20th Century Moses" as she committed herself to helping beleaguered Jews around the world, Ruth has seen more suffering than most of us could bear to witness. Below are just a few examples of her adventures and extraordinary courage:

- At 24, as an international correspondent for the *New York Herald Tribune*, Ruth was the first photojournalist to travel to and document the Soviet Arctic and Siberian labor camps, interviewing the prisoners and pioneers that survived Stalin.
- In 1941, at age 30, Ruth was appointed by U.S. Secretary of the Interior Harold L. Ickes as a field representative to the Alaska Territory where she took some of the earliest color photos of the Alaska region. She had to cover the territory by plane, truck and dogsled for 18 months to look into homesteading opportunities for G.I.s after World War II.
- In 1944, Ruth was assigned a covert mission by the Secretary

of the Interior to escort 1,000 Holocaust survivors from Italy to the U.S., the only Jews given refuge in this country during the war. President Roosevelt had given her the honorary rank of "general" so that she would not be killed if captured by the Nazis, just sent to a prisoner-of-war camp. She then fought for the refugees' citizenship once in the US and recorded this experience in her book *Haven* which became a musical play in 1993 and television mini-series in 2001.

- In 1947, a few thousand Holocaust survivors, including 600 orphans, were trying to enter Haifa on a boat, called the *S.S. Exodus 1947*, when they came under siege by the British who did not wish them to enter British-controlled Palestine. Ruth photographed the aftermath of the attack by the British and her images were published in *Life* magazine. She also reported the incident to the *Herald Tribune*. Ruth followed the people of the *Exodus 1947* and photographed them when they were herded onto three prison ships. She represented the entire American press aboard the ship *Runnymede Park*, documenting and photographing the refugees.

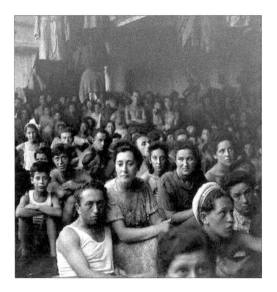

Holocaust survivors aboard the M.V. Runnymede Park, 1947, photographed by Ruth Gruber.

Ruth's reporting helped ensure the safety of thousands of Jews and her book, *Exodus 1947: The Ship That Launched a Nation,* was used as a source for the Leon Uris novel, *Exodus,* and the film by the same name.

For a total of thirty-two years as a correspondent, Ruth Gruber captured the triumph of the human spirit.

The world today

Over her lifetime, Ruth Gruber has written 19 books, all of which educate readers about injustices which she herself witnessed, eminent world figures such as Virginia Woolf, Ben Gurion and Golda Meir with whom she was closely acquainted, and her own personal journey through an extraordinary life.

REACHING 100 & BEYOND! 101 YEARS

Lifestyle

General health	Ruth was generally healthy, although she had gall bladder issues in her late 30s which she felt was due to her diet at the time.
Smoking	"Yes, I thought it would make me look older and taller. When I would look for an adjective, I would take a cigarette." She thought at the time it would help her creativity; however, she quit in her 30s.
Alcohol	Never, she wasn't interested in alcohol.
Nutrition	"Was very health-conscious after I had gall bladder problems. Growing up with a lot of chicken fat in my mother's cooking was a written guarantee to give you heartburn and gall bladder trouble. After I had my gall bladder removed at age 41, I consumed nothing fried and ate healthy foods." Ruth has always maintained a slender figure.

Physical activity	Nothing routinely; however, Ruth was always very active and for a time she "played ping pong avidly when in Alaska with the soldiers."
Current interests	Ruth continues to write, lecture and inspire others. When she was 90, she went on a 20-city tour to publicize the reprinting of four of her books.
Family	Ruth was married and widowed twice; she has been a widow for many years. She has two children and four grandchildren who live out of state.

Family history

	AGE OF DEATH	CAUSE OF DEATH
Mother	100	natural causes
Father	63	diabetes
Brother	64	heart attack
Brother	late 80s	natural causes
Brother	90s	natural causes
Sister	91	natural causes

What does Ruth think of the world today?
"Sad... our scientists have helped, but politically,
I am really concerned about the world."

Pediatrician, Co-Developer Of The Whooping Cough Vaccine

Born: February 1, 1898, in Portal, Georgia

Current residence: Athens, Georgia

DR. LEILA DENMARK

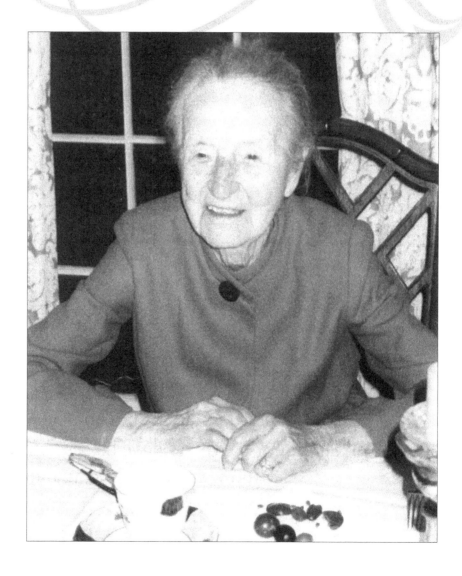

Words of Wisdom

114

"Eat right and do what you love. Whatever you love to do is play; doing what you don't like to do is work. I have never worked a day in my life!"

Dr. Leila Denmark is a world record holder in more ways than one. Before she retired at the age of 103, she was the oldest practicing pediatrician in the world. At age 114, she is the 4th oldest verified living person in the world. She also recently became one of the top 100 oldest people who ever lived.

Besides her extreme longevity, Leila lived an extraordinary existence saving countless lives.

In 1928, she graduated from the Medical College of Georgia. Remarkably, she was the only woman in her graduating class. Following her residency, Leila became the first physician at Henrietta Eggleston Hospital, a pediatric hospital that had just opened on the campus of Emory University. Following her work there, for the next 70+ years she practiced privately out of her home where she never

> "The greatest change I have seen in my life is the neglect of children. Pizza is going to support a whole generation of cardiologists!"

refused a patient, even those who could not pay.

A life devoted to saving children

Leila devoted much of her life to serving children and expressed her passionate views on child-rearing in her best-selling book, *Every Child Should Have a Chance,* published 40 years ago. She also wrote a book 30 years later, at age 104, titled *Dr. Leila Denmark Said It! Advice for Mothers from America's Most Experienced Pediatrician.*

A woman way ahead of her time, Leila was one of the first doctors to object to cigarette smoking around children and drug use in pregnant women. She said, "The greatest change I have seen in my life is the neglect of children."

Leila also had strong concerns about the nutrition of children. She believed that cow's milk was unhealthy [which is supported by current research as well—read the "China Study" by T. Colin Campbell]. She also repeatedly told children and their parents to eat whole fruits rather than fruit juices and to drink primarily water. Leila believed, "Pizza is going to

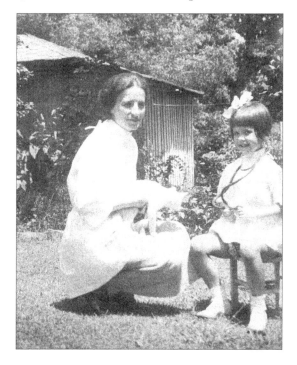

Leila with her daughter Mary. Courtesy of Mary Denmark Hutcherson.

support a whole generation of cardiologists!"

Sugar is the Devil

Leila certainly practiced what she preached. She drank only hot water every day—no coffee, tea, fruit juice, soft drinks, and absolutely no alcohol. She also avoided sugar like the plague. When she was a young adult, she developed arthritis. Until this day, Leila swears that cutting out sugar completely cured her arthritis. Even in her centenarian years, she refused cake on her birthday, as there was too much sugar in it.

"From *can* until *can't*"

According to Leila, "I would work from *can* until *can't*, beginning my office hours at 8 a.m., I would stay until the

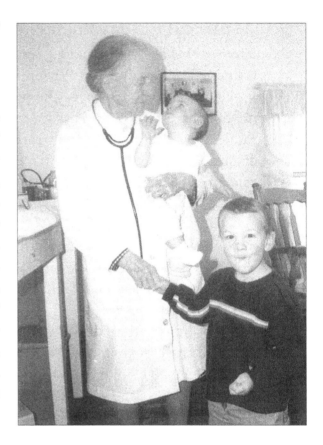

Dr. Denmark with patients in 2000. Courtesy of Mary Denmark Hutcherson

last patient left and I was available on any day at any hour." According to her daughter Mary, "Mother took as long as she needed to see each patient with no appointments needed and was exceedingly busy during WWII as many doctors were in the military. Additionally," she says, "during the Great Depression, she treated most patients without pay; she just loved what she did, she wasn't in it for the money."

A miraculous development

Mary said that her mother's greatest success was her work in developing the Pertussis (or Whooping Cough) vaccine that saved an untold number of lives over the past 75 years. However, according to Leila, her greatest success was each time she helped a child who came to her looking like "the wrath of God, and after a few months of good nutrition and medical treatment, if necessary, would blossom and bloom as a fine healthy child."

An anomaly in her great family

Born in Georgia, Leila was the third oldest of 12 siblings and the only one still living. Most of her siblings succumbed to heart disease and some to cancer. The youngest sibling to die was 25 years old and the oldest was 88.

According to Mary, there were a few significant differences between the lifestyle habits of her mother's siblings and Leila herself. Her siblings all smoked and drank regularly while Leila abhorred both. While they regularly ate pork fat from their family farm, Leila wouldn't dare touch it. And, while they all had their fair share of syrup and other sugar-laden substances, Leila essentially boycotted refined sugar for the majority of her life.

Valuable advice

Even after retiring at 103, Leila's phone was still constantly ringing as parents from all over Georgia sought out her unique and valuable advice on living a healthy and happy life. Here are some of her words of wisdom that Leila generously shared with her patients, their families and thousands of readers in her books:

- Avoid junk food
- Love what you do
- Drinking cow's milk is dangerous
- Treat others as you would like to be treated
- Avoid sugar

- A sense of humor is very important for longevity
- Children are not getting parental guidance and it's wrecking this nation
- We need to think about everything we eat and drink
- During the Great Depression, 11,000 of America's 25,000 banks closed, so save what you can, appreciate what you have
- As a doctor, it is important to find the root cause of a problem
- Never raise your hand or *your voice* to a child
- Parenting has gone out of style
- Children and adults should eat fruit instead of drinking fruit juices
- Drink only water.

Longevity is a pattern in all that she does. Leila married John Eustice Denmark and they were together for 62 years until his death at 91, just eleven years ago.

A national treasure, if you mention Dr. Leila Denmark's name anywhere in Georgia or to most anyone in the field of medicine, they will certainly be familiar with her incredible life and humanitarianism, and many were indeed one of her patients. There is even an exit named after her on a Georgia highway!

> NOTE: *As this super-centenarian has lost some of her memory, much of the information has been provided by her daughter Mary, who has lived with her for the past 7 years and has been close to her for her entire life.*

Lifestyle

Smoking	Never, "hated it with a passion."
Alcohol	Never, "hated it even worse."
Nutrition	Never had a weight problem. Enjoyed meat, green vegetables, and a starch for supper and an egg, toast and hot water for breakfast. She only drank hot water; no coffee, tea or soft drinks and often did not eat lunch, as she was busy working. She never ate sugar or dessert, except on occasion some honey on toast. On occasion when she ate out, she enjoyed shrimp and lobster.
Physical activity	No formal exercise but was on her feet most of the time, moving constantly. Even in her 90s, she walked to her fish pond each afternoon, which was a round trip of a half-mile. She seldom sat still and was always busy with something.
Current interests	After retiring, at 103, Leila Denmark still consulted with patients until 3 years ago. She enjoyed gardening, making her own clothes and reading until her vision slowly deteriorated. She traveled in her later years but always wanted to get back home. She also enjoys eating out and going back and forth to her house in Forsyth County for short visits.
Family	One daughter, with whom she lives, two grandsons, two great-grandchildren and several nieces and nephews who visit her regularly.

Family history

	AGE OF DEATH	CAUSE OF DEATH
Mother	45	cancer
Father	65	heart disease
Brother	88	heart disease
Sister	87	cancer
Brother	85	heart disease
Brother	75	heart disease
Brother	75	heart disease
Sister	72	heart disease
Sister	64	heart disease
Sister	55	cancer
Brother	54	heart disease
Brother	51	heart disease
Sister	25	heart disease

Note: *Six of Leila Denmark's nieces and nephews also died of heart disease, all under the age of 60.*

After retiring at 103, Leila's phone was still constantly ringing as parents sought out her unique and valuable advice.

Professional Singer, Dental Assistant, Matriarch
Born: July 25, 1904, in St. Louis, Illinois
Current residence: Rancho Palos Verdes, California

BONITA ZIGRANG

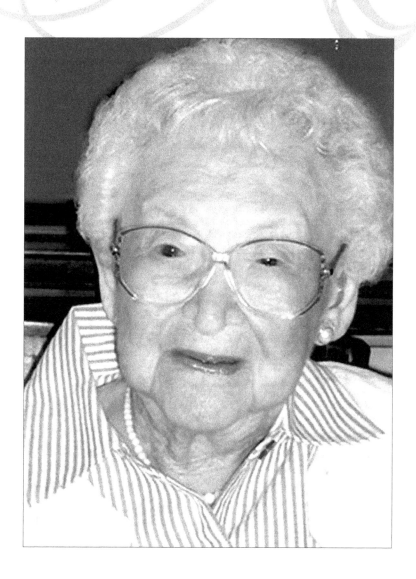

108 Words of Wisdom

"Have a good appetite,

lots of friends,

and keep busy."

I heard about this lovely 108-year-old woman over a year ago through a friend who discovered her on Facebook! As I was looking for vibrant extreme elders for this book, it seemed that Bonita Zigrang's contemporary attitude might just fit the bill.

On her Facebook page, she was boldly requesting visitors to "friend" her as she wanted to see how many friends she could accumulate by her 107th birthday. Given how charming an idea this was, coupled with the networking impact of Facebook, it was not surprising that Bonita soon accumulated over 1,200 friends!

Although it turned out that this audacious endeavor was in fact initiated by one of her grandsons, I definitely wanted to find out more about this mysterious woman and to learn how she got to be so very old.

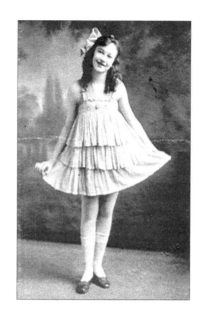

Bonita in her early years, singing and dancing. Photo courtesy of the Zigrangs

A singing career at a young age was launched to support her family

Although Bonita recently suffered a stroke, at 108 years old she is still sharp as a tack. She still lives independently in a multi-level house and until she was 98, had no assistance.

When Bonita was only 6 years old, her father died from an accidental fall. He was working at the World's Fair at the time. In order to help support her mother, Bonita and her sisters left school and started singing. Bonita left in the 10th grade and obtained her first job singing in Remix's Music Store. Her friend would play the piano and Bonita sang the sheet music in order to sell it. They both did the bookkeeping for Mr. Remix as well. Bonita recalls, "A woman I knew who worked across the street, and had the same job as me, got pregnant by the owner of the store. His name was Mr. Cooper. Their son became a famous actor, Jackie Cooper."

Besides Remix's Music Store, Bonita would perform outside of Ferris wheels, carousels and various clubs and, on one occasion, performed with a band at a lake in a park. This is where she met her husband at age 24. "He was working as a

In their 20s, Bonita and Margaret King were professional singers throughout southern California.

canoe pusher to make extra money while he was in dental school. It was love at first sight."

Bonita's most satisfying time in her career was when she was singing with Margaret King (of the King Sisters). In their 20s, Bonita and Margaret King were professional singers throughout southern California; they were on the Orpheum circuit. They were also the opening act at the Balboa Theatre in San Diego.

Just recently, Bonita was invited to the rebirth of the Balboa Theatre. She was 104 when she went to the re-dedication and was acknowledged for her part during its original launch.

Loving life in her platinum years

Following her singing career, Bonita worked at her husband's dental office for many years. They lived at the time in the neighborhood of Watts, Los Angeles during the time of the dangerous, racially-driven riots in 1965. The family convinced them to move closer to them in Rancho Palos Verdes so that they would be safer. Given that 34 people died in those riots and there was more than $40 million dollars in property damage, the family was thankful that their parents got out of there unscathed.

Bonita was in her 70s when her husband passed away and she continued to work there until her son Richard (who took over the practice) realized that she needed to finally relax and convinced her to retire.

> "We went on a cruise when she was about 97 and we lost her for about an hour. When we finally found her, she was at a bar happily drinking a Bloody Mary!"
> – Dr. Richard Zigrang (Bonita's son)

Bonita had a large circle of friends until she "outlived them all." She loved to travel with other seniors as well as her family.

According to Richard Zigrang, "We went on a cruise when she was about 97 and we lost her for about an hour. When we finally found her, she was at a bar happily drinking a Bloody Mary! She was traveling until as recent as last year, always eager to go with the family overseas or down the Mississippi."

Bonita was always very involved with her family. She took care of her mother who lived with her until she died at 91. She would also often stay with her sister-in-law who was older than she. As she got older, she mostly stayed home and took care of the house, which she absolutely treasured.

Bonita still loves to read and when she started to lose her sight, she didn't let that stop her. Bonita ordered books with Braille and purchased a machine to magnify the words. She also enjoys frequent visits from her rather large extended family that simply adore her.

"She just loves listening to all of their stories," says Richard Zigrang. Although she had said that she worried about money, her son said that it was unnoticeable, as she just never complained.

According to her family, one thing is very noticeable—Bonita still keeps on singing.

REACHING 100 & BEYOND! 108 YEARS

Lifestyle

General health	Bonita led a clean life and never had a serious illness except for a bout with gastritis and a hysterectomy. She has poor vision now and recently had a stroke which left her unable to walk.
Smoking	Never.
Alcohol	Very infrequent.

Nutrition	Bonita says she didn't have a regimented diet but was never overweight. "We ate whatever we had." She cooked and ate out frequently.
Physical activity	No regular physical activity.
Current interests	Singing, reading, housekeeping, traveling extensively.
Family	Bonita never remarried after her husband's death over 30 years ago. They were married just under 50 years and had 2 sons and a legacy of 9 grandchildren and 12 great-grandchildren. Bonita cherishes her time with her extended family that visits her 2 to 3 times per week.

Family history

	AGE OF DEATH	CAUSE OF DEATH
Mother	91	natural causes
Father	77	accident
Sister	90	stroke
Sister	50	cancer

On *Facebook* she accumulated 1,200 friends by her 107th birthday.

Former NBA Player, Teacher, Insurance Salesman
Born: September 6, 1913, in Newark, New Jersey
Current residence: Tavares, Florida

BENJAMIN GOLDFADEN

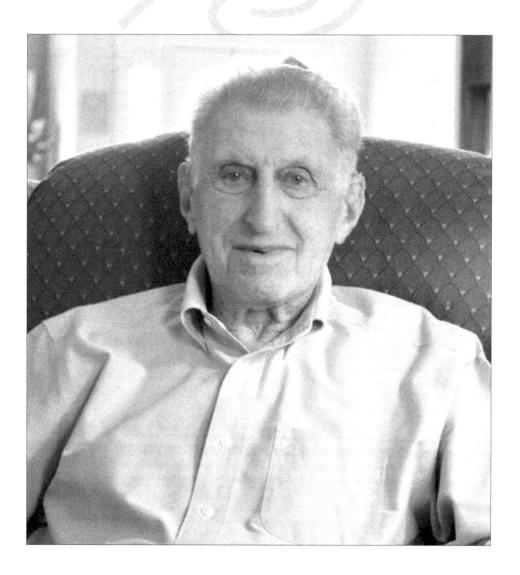

Words of Wisdom

99

"Stay active... even at 100. Eat in a balanced way... Don't stay mad at anything—you have to get used to the losses, otherwise you can't win. Lastly, stay close with your family, they keep you thinking."

I met Benjamin Goldfaden in his lovely home in South Florida that he shares with his adoring daughter and son-in-law. He is a lofty 6-foot-1-inches, well built, sharp as a tack with a wonderful sense of humor—it was incredibly hard to believe that this man was nearly 100. It was not surprising however that he had been a professional basketball player.

How to get through a crisis: play ball

Benjamin's family fled to America from Russia and Germany on the brink of WWI. Most of the extended family was able to escape; but some were not as fortunate. The Goldfadens settled in Newark, New Jersey. Prudently, many of the fellow Jewish immigrants in their community created an "insurance fund" to help those in

> "I loved going to the sweat baths with my father and his friends as a young child. Only men were allowed and they often brought us kids along with them."

the community who may need assistance in the future. Each family contributed about 5 cents per week.

Many years later, this insurance fund came in handy for young Benjamin as his father unexpectedly died of a brain tumor in his 40s. Tragically, he left Benjamin and his 4 siblings with only their mom to raise them during the Great Depression. Benjamin was only 14, the year after he became a Bar Mitzvah.

He fondly remembered his dad: "I loved going to the sweat baths with my father and his friends as a young child. Only men were allowed (no women) and they often brought us kids along with them."

Many Russian Jewish immigrants in New York, who were often trapped in tenements with no baths and worked in sweatshops, patronized bathhouses owned by the more fortunate immigrants. The Russian bath provided a social center.

When I asked how they were able to manage, Benjamin described how his close-knit community helped out as well as his relatives. He was relinquished to selling watermelons on the street for a time and he and his brother started paper routes while in high school. However, he said that he felt unaffected by the crisis as his focus and passion was always on playing ball.

In high school, he quickly made varsity basketball as a freshman and his skills grew by leaps and bounds. He didn't do much of anything else but play ball, also dabbling in football, baseball and tennis. In 1937, he won a full scholarship to George Washington University for basketball. "I left

> "I left [for George Washington University] with $20 to my name."

with $20 to my name, which my sister had given to me as she was the only one working at the time." He went on to obtain his Masters Degree at GW in Administration and Education.

Love, segregation & pro basketball

While at GW, Benjamin experienced the tribulations of anti-Semitism, even from his own teammates. He joined a Jewish fraternity to feel more accepted. As his popularity grew as an athlete, the anti-Semitism waned. Shortly after, Benjamin met the love of his life, Libby, married her, and they were blissfully wed for 68 years. Deprecatingly, he quips, "This was fortunate for me as she was a hell of a lot smarter and helped with some of my classes. It was the best thing that ever happened to me." When asked his secret to staying married for so long, he responded, "My wife was the exact opposite of me. She was very literate and I was a jock. We were a good balance." His eyes well up. "I think about her every night."

> "My wife was the exact opposite of me. She was very literate and I was a jock. We were a good balance." His eyes well up. "I think about her every night."

In 1937, while at GW, Benjamin was drafted by Heurich Brewery in the District of Columbia for their semi-pro basketball team (the Brewers) which quickly moved to pro status. Benjamin made $25 a game playing twice a week. When the Brewers joined the newly formed ABA league, his salary "soared" to $40 per game. However, when WWII commenced, Heurich had to disband the team.

In 1940, Benjamin was transferred to a team in Harrisburg, which also disbanded eventually due to the war. He was transferred one more time until, at age 31, he was drafted into the Navy for 2 years. What did he do in the Navy? "We played basketball!" Luckily,

> ## "I recall only 2 black teams then, the Renaissance and the Globetrotters."

the war ended just before he was to be transferred overseas. Baltimore's ABA team drafted him right out of the Navy and then transferred him to Trenton. They figured that Benjamin, a Jersey boy, would attract many spectators to the game. And, he did.

As stadiums were scarce in those days, Benjamin and his team played mostly in dancehalls, where spectators would dance following the games. While professional sports were watched by all ethnic groups, the teams were strictly segregated with the all-white teams playing against some all-black teams. "I recall only two black teams then, the Renaissance and the Globetrotters."

When the NBA league was formed in 1946, Red Auerbach, who was coaching the Washington Capitols, immediately drafted Benjamin. [Auerbach later became president of the Boston Celtics.] Benjamin was elated; however, he only could play a few games as he was working as a physical education teacher to support his wife and two children and couldn't leave his job to commit full time to the sport. "The other players

> ## "I was the oldest person on the team at 33."

had just graduated so they had the freedom to commit. I was the oldest person on the team at 33." Unfortunately, that was the end of his basketball career. He gave up between $2,000 and $5,000 per year, the going rate in the late-1940s.

A town built by Eleanor Roosevelt

For nearly 50 years, Benjamin lived and worked in a newly-formed public cooperative community now known as "Old Greenbelt", in Maryland. He worked as a recreational director, physical education teacher, and as an insurance salesman until he retired at 65.

In 1953 Old Greenbelt was one of three towns in the country that was developed with the assistance of Eleanor Roosevelt. The US government was attempting to foster a "utopian" community that would be practical while easing the critical housing shortage. The new community provided affordable housing for federal workers who qualified based on their income and willingness to become active in the community.

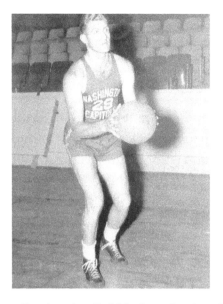

Benjamin Goldfaden playing for the NBA Washington Capitols in 1946. Photo courtesy Benjamin Goldfaden

Benjamin's wife Libby had worked as a psychiatric social worker for the Veteran's Association so fortunately they qualified. The Goldfadens raised three children while both worked full-time. They took different shifts, one caring for the children while the other worked. Thriving in this close-knit community, Benjamin was inducted into the Washington, DC area Hall of Fame for softball and was on the board of directors at Prince George's Community College.

Creating a playground in his later years

As soon as they both retired, Benjamin and Libby moved to Florida. They met a wonderful group of friends and continued their pulsating life of social and physical activity, spending lots of time with family. Benjamin has lost his wife and most of his friends, but continues to meet new friends through his children.

How does he see the world today? "I thought the world was tough back then, but the way the world is looking now reminds me that the human race is very stupid! We just keep repeating the same mistakes."

The obvious question at the time, *what do you think of Jeremy Lin?* "I think he is a good player, not a great player, and will be in trouble because of all the publicity. He used to have room to breathe and did some great things. Now that everyone is onto him, his opponents are all over him and he's already not doing as well." Words of wisdom from a man who has been in those star shoes.

Benjamin describes himself as an "easy-going, quiet fellow who never raises hell," although he can be "quite impatient at times."

REACHING FOR 100 & BEYOND! 99 YEARS

Lifestyle

General health	Benjamin was exceptionally healthy most of his life but has weathered some severe storms in his later years. At 70, he had an abdominal aneurysm that was successfully treated; at 91 he had a triple bypass. At 88, he broke his arm and hip (playing racquetball). "He just never slows down," says his family, and is never content to sit for long.
Smoking	Never.
Alcohol	Never.
Nutrition	Benjamin has worked on maintaining a lean 180 lb. frame his entire life. He was never overweight. Growing up during the Depression, he learned a culture of moderation. As he got older, he watched his diet, consuming small meals of chicken, lamb or fish with vegetables, lots of fruit, starch and red meat on occasion. He consumes sweets occasionally and has never taken vitamins.

Physical activity	Extremely active since he was a child. Besides basketball, he was active in football, softball and tennis. In his retirement years in Florida, he swam, played golf, and became an avid racquetball player. He still walks regularly.
Current interests	Watching sports, time with family, reading the paper cover to cover, playing poker, going to the racetrack (dog and horses).
Family	Lived with his wife in their own home until she died 6 years ago. Now living with his daughter, Vicky, and son-in-law, Dennis, in a lovely, warm home in a gated rural community in Florida. He has three children, 10 grandchildren, and 13 great-grandchildren, many of them living somewhat close by.

Family history

	AGE OF DEATH	CAUSE OF DEATH
Mother	late 80s	natural causes
Father	40s	brain tumor
Sister	90s	natural causes
Brother	70	heart disease
Sister	70s	heart disease
Brother	60s	heart attack (heavy drinker and smoker)

Benjamin is a lofty 6-foot-1-inches and sharp as a tack.

Professional Golfer (last surviving member of the 1st Masters)

Born: November 14, 1910, in Bangor, Wales

Current residence: Stuart, Florida

SAMUEL 'ERRIE' BALL

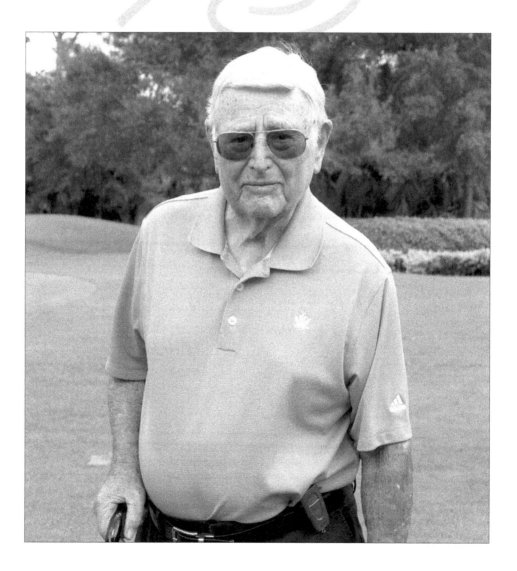

102 Words of Wisdom

"Have a good wife,
two scotches a night,
and be easy-going."

I met Errie Ball and his lovely wife, Maxie, at the beautiful Willoughby Golf Club in Stuart, Florida, where he taught golf for over 20 years. At Willoughby sits a proud bronze statue of Errie and on the walls, numerous media clippings and letters from fans ranging from Arnold Palmer to George W. Bush. Errie remains Willoughby's pro emeritus. However, the term emeritus should be used lightly as Errie, at 102, still manages to give some tips now and then. Indeed, fans from all over the country still travel to see Errie, hoping to receive advice that will transform their game.

Errie, sporting a crisp blue golf shirt, was charming and humorous with an irresistible British accent and sharp as a tack. Although Maxie did remind him about a thing or two!

A remarkable golfer and teacher

Born in Bangor, Wales, Errie's remarkable golf career started when he was just a teen. He was the youngest contestant ever to play in the British Open at 15 years of age in 1926. The winner of that tournament was the legendary Bobby Jones.

Errie came from a family of golfers. His dad, a pro in England, taught him the game early on. He assisted his father, but moved to the United States at 20 to work as an assistant pro under his uncle, Frank Ball, at the East Lake Golf Club in Atlanta, GA. His brother was also a pro in England and is still playing, well into his 90s and his sister, 97, always loved the game as well.

> "My most memorable golf moment was when Bobby Jones invited me to play in the first Masters Tournament, in 1934."

While Errie was working in Atlanta, Bobby Jones had started mentoring him and Errie built quite a reputation as a golfer. According to Errie, "My most memorable golf moment was when Bobby Jones invited me to play in the 1st Masters Tournament, then called the Augusta National Invitational Tournament, in 1934."

Errie and 71 other players were invited to this momentous event. The players stayed at the Bon Air Vanderbilt hotel for the special rate of $5 per night including breakfast, lunch and dinner. Errie finished the tournament in a tie for 38th place. He is the last surviving member of those 72 men.

After his tour, Errie moved up to head professional at a country club in Mobile, Alabama. His tenure there ended prematurely when he served in the Navy for 4 years during World War II.

Following his military service, Errie played in the winter tour and then accepted another job as a pro in Chicago for several years.

Due to his accomplishments there, Errie was inducted into the Illinois Golf Hall of Fame in 1990.

Although he didn't play in the Masters again until 1957, Errie, in his long career as a club professional, qualified for nearly 40 tournaments including 20 US Opens.

When I asked about the difference in the PGA now versus 80 years ago, Errie recalls, "a golf pro in those days not only had to be a good player, he had to be a good club maker because we had to make our own clubs and sell them as well." He learned the craft from his father and Uncle Frank. His favorite clubs now? Wilson.

Who is the best player nowadays? "McIlroy is moving up but he still has to knock Tiger off of his seat. Tiger is always in there. He has a very fine golf swing and has so much experience, he's not afraid of winning."

Best player ever? "Bobby Jones, Sam Snead, Byron Nelson in that order."

Did Errie ever get a hole-in-one? "I got two hole-in-ones in the same round when I played in Chicago."

Handicap? "Scratch" [a zero handicap].

Low score? "62 in Tuscon, Arizona."

Advice for the young golfers? Errie quips, "Practice hard and drink two Scotches every night." He jokes but he has been doing that every day for many decades!

Still playing? "I played up until 2 years ago when I started to lose my balance. It wouldn't be good to be swinging my club with no balance!"

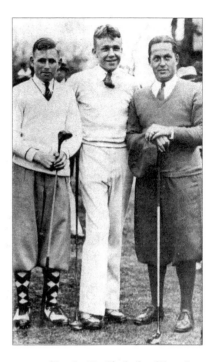

Errie Ball, left, Charles Yates, center, with host Bobby Jones at the Masters Tournament in 1934. Photo courtesy of Willoughby Country Club

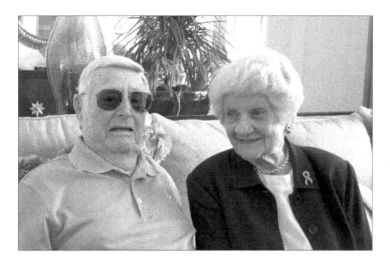

Errie Ball, 102, and his wife, Maxwell (Maxie), 97.

A shipboard romance

Errie met his wife Maxie in 1936 while he was on a ship returning from England after a British Open tournament. Both Errie and Maxie were engaged to others at the time, but not for long. "It was a shipboard romance. She was returning to her hometown of Virginia after a European vacation. The ship landed in New York. I went back to Alabama, where I was working at the time, and she to Virginia. We corresponded by letters and phone and soon after, got married." Errie and Maxie, 97, have been married for 76 years and still live in their own home with the aid of a nurse. His secret to a long, wonderful marriage: "Don't ever go to bed with nasty thoughts in your mind and you will have a happy marriage."

Errie describes his personality as just "nice" and Maxie added "and easy-going." During the Great Depression, while he was a head pro in Alabama, everyone, including him, lost a lot of money, but that didn't deter him from following his true passion and pressing on.

Errie said he would love to be remembered as "a good golf pro and teacher." And, he just may be getting his wish. Last year, Errie, to his humble surprise, was inducted into the PGA Hall of Fame.

> "Don't ever go to bed with nasty thoughts in your mind and you will have a happy marriage."

102 YEARS

Lifestyle

General health	Errie was healthy his entire life until he reached his 90s when he developed some heart issues. He is dealing with a faulty equilibrium following a fall. He walks with a cane he mistakens for a five-iron.
Smoking	Yes, but gave it up 70 years ago after the Navy.
Alcohol	Oh, yes. Errie drinks 2 Scotches every night!
Nutrition	Errie eats "generally healthy, vegetables, mostly fish and sometimes a steak. I tend to avoid fatty and fried foods, but I do sometimes eat bacon and eggs for breakfast. I sometimes miss lunch as well. I eat home-cooked meals and eat out as well."
Physical activity	Errie was always very active playing golf and giving lessons. He was never obese, but has been 10 to 20 lbs. overweight at times.
Current interests	Errie played golf and taught regularly until he was 100. Per a source at Willoughby, he continues to give golf tips to people from all over the country, sometimes from his golf cart and checks his fan mail nearly every day at the club.
Family	Errie and Maxie have one daughter in Miami who they see regularly, and two grandchildren.

Family History

	AGE OF DEATH	CAUSE OF DEATH
Mother	90s	natural causes
Father	90s	natural causes
Brother	early 80s	not available
Sister	n/a	living, age 97 (Africa)
Brother	n/a	living, age 90s (England)

Life Insurance Agent

Born: May 19, 1916, in Chicago, Illinois

Current residence: Hermosa Beach, California

ALYSE LAEMMLE

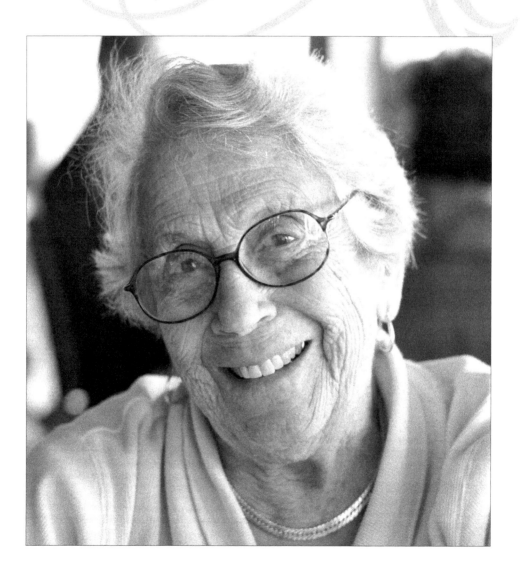

Words of Wisdom

96

"Never run out of responsibility; if you don't have one, find one. Find a cause and knock yourself out for it. It will enhance your brainpower, interest in life, and keep you alive longer. I'm alert because I work. Virtue is its own reward."

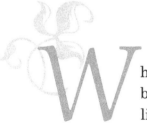

When I first met Alyse, I was instantly touched by her enthusiasm, sense of humor and passion for life.

A quick and nimble learner

Exceptionally sharp at 96, it was no surprise when Alyse apprised me that she graduated high school at age 15, and Northwestern University at 19. When I asked how she skipped 2 years of school, she responded, "I was a bright student and in those days, they didn't know what to do with the smart kids, so they would just skip us. However, nobody ever bothered to teach me the multiplication tables. Arithmetic and I are not on a friendly basis."

Following graduation, Alyse's mother sent her to study in

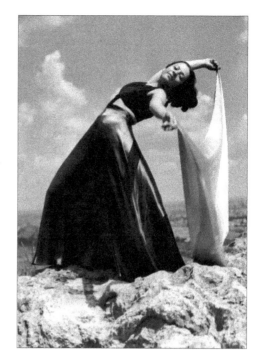

Alyse practicing dance in Hungary.
Photo courtesy of Ms. Laemmle

Budapest where she studied dance under a remarkable teacher and dancer for a year. She studied for 7 to 8 hours a day dancing and learning dance theory. When she returned to the States, she taught dance for a few years and performed professionally, singing and dancing for years even after she met her beloved husband, Kurt.

From riches to rags

A new chapter opened for Alyse after she married Kurt. She was thrust into the exciting, but volatile motion picture industry. Kurt and his brother operated five motion picture studios, and one of Kurt's relatives, Carl Laemmle, was the sole owner of Universal Pictures and a very wealthy man. Alyse recalled, "We used to go to his enormous estate for barbeques. I remember the time he gave out over 600 affidavits for Jews to immigrate from Germany during WWII."

"My husband's business was phenomenal until the invention of television. The brothers didn't take television seriously

"I never knew how rich we were until we were poor."

until it was too late. At the time (in the late 1940s), it destroyed the motion picture theatres one by one. I never knew how rich we were until we were poor."

It took 6 long years for the Laemmles to pay off their debts as Kurt strongly believed in paying back every penny personally, rather than declaring bankruptcy.

Alyse admitted it was one of the most challenging times of her life.

Every blessing starts with a "schlamazel"

After these years, Alyse became an advocate for those who were less fortunate. She was a volunteer for the United Jewish Appeal (UJA) for eleven years, speaking as vice chairman of the National Women's Division

"Losing our money enabled me to get my job as a life insurance agent, which for me is a way of life filled with love and loyalty!"

all over the country. She would have become national chairman if she didn't have to get a paying job. She explains, "Kurt's insurance agent, our friend, took me to lunch one day and told me all about families whose lives were saved by life insurance and those who went down the drain who didn't have any. After that, I would have hocked my soul to be an agent. I lost 12 pounds during training as I was so excited by what I was going to do. My first boss taught me that the secret of selling was to really listen, ask questions, don't lecture, just listen."

In those days, prestigious life insurance companies didn't hire women, but given that both Kurt and Alyse eventually teamed up as partners, were the first husband and wife team ever to become Chartered Life Underwriter's and were both life members of the Million Dollar Round Table, Alyse was the first woman ever accepted to one of the most illustrious insurance companies in the country, Mass Mutal, where she has been for 52 years and counting.

"I strongly believe that all of the main blessings in life start with a *schlamazel*," which Laemmle described as a Yiddish word relating to bad luck. "Losing our money pushed me to get my job as a life insurance agent, which for me, is a way of life filled with love and loyalty—it's just wonderful!"

After 62 years as an agent, Alyse is still working long days and sometimes nights from her beautiful home just yards from the Pacific Ocean. She says, "I really love this stuff I peddle."

> "I'm not an idiot, I know that I am close to the day when I'm going to die. But it feels pretty darn good to know that I've used my life the way I have."

Loving life at 96

"Here I am at 96," Alyse states with enthusiasm. "I am never lonely, never bored. I'm always busy, surrounded by people who care about me, all because I am an insurance agent. I'm so involved in my clients' lives."

She continues passionately, "I'm never going to retire as long as I am competent. I take the word service very seriously. This will be one of the best years I've ever had in business and I haven't had to look for business in 45 years."

Alyse describes how her clients, although many have moved away, still retain her as their agent. However, she adds, "I'm not an idiot, I know that I am close to the day when I'm going to die. But it feels pretty darn good to know that I've used my life the way I have."

Alyse describes herself as an incurable optimist who is not a worrier. And, although she has been cheated a few times in the past, she truly believes that 95% of the people in the world are good.

"Most important thing in my life will always be my husband. Advice? Pick a good human being, someone you like even more than you love."

Charity and poetry

What was the most important thing in Alyse's life? "My husband." Advice? "Pick a good human being, someone you like even more than you love. Kurt was very charitable—even when he lost the money, he still managed to keep his annual pledges to charities."

Alyse and her husband were always charitable. "Charitable giving was always the core of our lives." She gives frequently to The Innocence Project, an organization that helps exonerate innocent people from jail and attempts to repair the systematic failings of the justice system. Another favorite charity of Alyse's is Goodwill, which recently gave her the Benefactor of the Year award for generously contributing for over 50 years.

The Laemmles were married for 57 years until Kurt died in 1994. She says, "Even 18 years after his passing, I still have a crush on him!"

Besides her years as a speaker for the United Jewish Appeal, Alyse is also a poet. Her words speak volumes about how she lives her life, and has been living it for so many years. I will leave you with one of Alyse's free verse poems, published in her synagogue community calendar after she turned 95:

If I Could Live My Life Again

Now that my 95th birthday has
  come and gone, I wonder
  what I'd do differently if I
  could live my life again.
I was born in a generation
  when parents dictated and
  children obeyed, but this
  resulted in a grown-up-me
  with no sense of self.
I now believe growing-up
  years need to combine
  learning from personal
  mistakes with credit for
  personal successes.
So, if I could be a child again
  I'd try to think for myself
  whenever this made sense.
  Then, sometimes I'd say
  'no.'

I'd have married the same man
  and loved him totally, those
  same 57 years.
I'd have listened and talked,
  cooked and baked...
  and loved him, but I'd
  appreciate him more.

I would have parented
  differently. I worked hard at
  chores no one remembers,
I made jam, baked cookies,
  packed super school
  lunches, but my daughters
  remember the lullabies I
  sang to them at bedtime
  and that I read to them
  from story books.
If I could be their young mom
  all over again, we'd sing
  lots more songs together

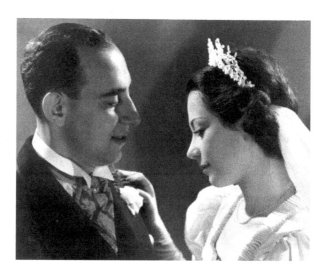

*Alyse and Kurt on
their wedding day.
Photo courtesy of Alyse
Laemmle*

70

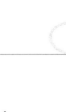

and we'd "waste" hours at
home, in playgrounds, at
the beach having fun.
We'd learn a lot and we'd all
grow up.

This time around, I worked
hard to succeed, to
accomplish more, to do
things better.
Next time I'd take more time
and thought searching for
meanings.
I've learned that sometimes
"less is more" and joy
comes from relating to
others.
My life's greatest treasure is
surely the love I receive,
and can give.

This time around, I worried
about lots of things. I rarely
reached the goals I set.
Next time I'd be patient with
my shortcomings.
Now old me is at peace with
myself and this brightens
up my days.

Is all this talk about living life
over a waste of time?
We all know this can't be, but
I can maximize each day I
still have left to live.
I believe this means giving in
every way, the most that I
can give,
Continuing some meaningful
work each day listening
to others... with my heart
engaged, treasuring, every
minute, this gift of my
life, thanking God for the
incredible world we were
given... for the glory of
sun, moon, stars, ocean,
sky, birds, trees, people,
and puppy dogs.

I think if I hold all this
gratitude and awe close to
my heart, I may get to live,
live, live until the day I die.

—*Alyse Laemmle,*
June 25, 2011

Lifestyle

General health	"My overall health is indecently well." Alyse takes no medication except one for a minor thyroid issue. She's never had any serious illnesses, has good hearing, an incredibly sharp wit and cognitive ability.
Smoking	Never.
Alcohol	Occasional glass of wine, no hard liquor.
Nutrition	"I love to cook and I cooked very fancy meals while married. I don't eat junk food. I prefer salads, thick soups, veggies, lots of chicken, red meat on occasion, and I should eat more fish. I try not to have a lot of carbs and almost never eat dessert. I watch what I eat and don't over-eat but I was always overweight." She takes multivitamins, 1000 mg C, calcium and coated aspirin for prevention.
Physical activity	"I'm not an athlete; however, I danced in my earlier years and went cycling 25 miles a day for a long while." In her golden years, she walked the beach with her dogs until her knees got bad and now exercises on a step machine.
Current interests	Alyse loves to cook for others. She enjoys giving money to various causes, donating 1/3 of her earned income, which is an important reason she continues to work.

Family	Alyse has 2 daughters, 5 grandchildren and 4 great-grandchildren. She sees one daughter who lives locally every other week, and one granddaughter "lives in her guest quarters."

Family history

	AGE OF DEATH	CAUSE OF DEATH
Mother	97	natural causes
Father	84	unknown
Sister	84	skin cancer

I was instantly touched
by her enthusiasm, sense of humor
and passion for life.

The World's Oldest Active Investment Professional
Born: December 19, 1905, in Manhattan, New York
Current residence: Manhattan, New York

IRVING KAHN

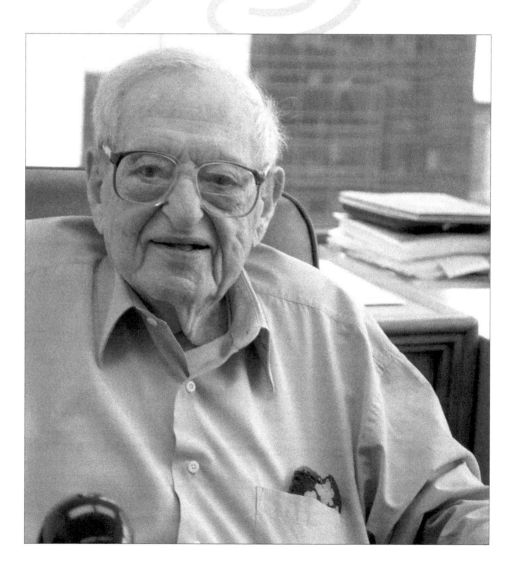

Words of Wisdom

106

*"It is very important
to have a widespread
curiousity about life."*

I discovered this remarkable man and his family of centenarians while perusing the cover of *New York Magazine*. The cover story was about a comprehensive study called the Longevity Genes Project, which took place at the Albert Einstein College of Medicine in New York. Dr. Nir Barzilai, the Director for the Institute of Aging, initiated this study in 1998 to determine whether centenarians had a common type of "longevity gene." His hope was to identify a gene or multiple genes that could lead to new drug therapies to help people live longer, and avoid or delay diseases such as cardiovascular, cancer, type 2 diabetes and Alzheimer's.

Irving and his three siblings all participated in this project along with over 500 subjects, aged 95 to 122 and their children. All of the older subjects, including the Kahn family, were deemed

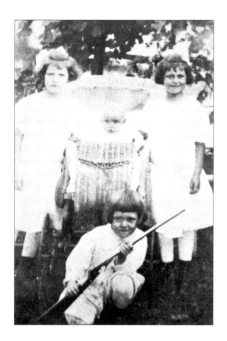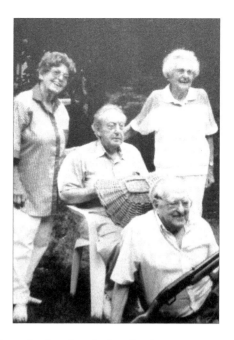

Kahn Family in the early 1900s (left photo) and also in their platinum years (right photo) at Peter's Connecticut home (left to right Happy, Peter, Lee and Irving (brandishing his rifle). Photos courtesy of Irving Kahn

"Super Agers" as they reached their extreme longevity never having experienced any of the above major diseases. Interestingly, Barzilai searched for genes that helped prevent disease in contrast to previous research focused on genes more likely to cause disease. Thus far, the results have been promising. Barzilai has indeed found common genes amongst some of the "Super Agers", including the Kahns, that may have contributed to their longevity and is already working on the development of new drug therapies.

Irving's siblings included Helen, a former talk-show host nicknamed "Happy" who died recently at 109; Leonore or "Lee," a noted humanitarian who died at 102 in 2005; and younger sibling, Peter, a former Hollywood photographer and cinematographer who is currently 102 and living in Connecticut with his wife. Unfortunately, Peter became blind about 5 years ago. The Kahns were at one time considered the world's oldest siblings.

> Dr. Barzilai had indeed found common genes amongst some of the "Super Agers."

Still working at 106, Irving Kahn was an ideal candidate for *Extraordinary Centenarians in America.* He agreed to meet with me in his office on the 22nd floor overlooking Madison Avenue where he still works 5 days a week.

A start in finance during the Great Depression

A soft-spoken, remarkably alert man with large reading glasses and new hearing aids, Irving vividly recalled his early childhood over 100 years ago. He recalled that his family of Eastern European Jews lived in Harlem, a neighborhood filled with immigrants from all over Europe. "Hungarians, Russians, Polish, I was exposed to many different people and languages early on." Perhaps this exposure incited his widespread curiosity about life and his thirst for learning. However, out of all his interests, from solar technology to aerospace, Irving's passion was always finance.

Irving decided not to finish his courses at City College. Why? He was presented with a coveted opportunity to work as a teaching assistant at Columbia Business School alongside perhaps the greatest investor of all time, Benjamin Graham. Benjamin Graham was considered to be the "father of security analysis and value investing." His textbooks are still considered to be required reading for most investors. One of Graham's most famous students... Mr. Warren Buffett.

Benjamin Graham became Irving's mentor and had such a profound influence on his life that Irving named one of his three

> "It was a rich man's business in those days and it was certainly anti-Jewish. Benjamin Graham gave Jewish kids a chance; he gave Jews an opportunity to get in. The [financial] industry is very different now."

sons after him, Thomas Graham. Irving says, "I think most people model their behavior by people they admire tremendously. It was a rich man's business in those days and it was certainly anti-Jewish. Benjamin Graham gave Jewish kids a chance; he gave Jews an opportunity to get in. The [financial] industry is very different now."

> Although currently son Thomas runs the business, which has about $700 million under management, Irving, the chairman, still works 5 to 6 hours every weekday and sits in the spacious corner office.

He then pointed to a photo of an oil painting of Graham commissioned by Buffett. This photo was squeezed in amongst several others pinned to his corkboard, most of them exhibiting his pride in life, his family.

Irving began his career in 1928, less than a year before the start of the Great Depression. Although you may think that quite unfortunate, Irving made very wise choices and had become a very successful man.

The 106-year-old chairman

Irving founded his current investment company, Kahn Brothers Group, Inc., with two of his sons, Thomas and Alan, in 1978. Although currently Thomas runs the business, which has about $700 million under management, Irving, the chairman, still works 5 to 6 hours every weekday and occupies the spacious corner office. Irving is still very involved in the firm's investments and reviews many of the investment decisions with Thomas.

On his desk sits a computer and two of his favorite newspapers, *The Wall Street Journal* and the *Financial Times*. He apprised me that his favorite read is *The Economist*, which he used to have shipped over from England "for two and a half dollars." Back then, he

"It is important to read non-fiction and continue to learn and explore. This keeps you young and mentally alert."

would relentlessly encourage *The Economist*'s publisher to start distributing the magazine in the US, which they eventually did. Irving chortled, "now they sell more issues here than they ever did in England."

Humble pie and so diversified

During our interview, Irving continuously stressed how vital it is to help people around you, to have diverse interests and a widespread curiosity. He passionately described his enormous library filled with books in his New York City home. "It is important to read non-fiction and continue to learn and explore. This keeps you young and mentally alert. Use your libraries."

He spoke of the progression of women during WWII. "As men were going to war and taken away from their jobs, suddenly women were needed to fill their spots. They learned to type as well as other skills for positions that were previously unavailable to them." This reminded Irving of his beloved wife, Ruth, a very educated woman with whom he was wed for 69 years. Ruth died 11 years ago.

According to his staff, Irving is extremely humble. One staffer quipped, "in the midst of a conversation outside of the office building, Mr. Kahn said, 'I have to run, the bus is here,' as he literally ran to catch the bus. Even in his late 90s, Mr. Kahn often rode the bus to and from work. He could have owned the bus." In 2003, a major blackout occurred throughout Manhattan. As the elevators were not in service, Irving had to walk down 22 flights of stairs. It was after

"Even in his late 90s, Mr. Kahn often rode the bus to and from work. He could have owned the bus."

> *He describes his personality as "going with the tide although my tide is different."*

that incident that his legs began to fail, relegating him to a walker and eventually a wheelchair.

Like most of the centenarians in this book, Irving does not bemoan life's challenges nor does he dwell on the past. He describes his personality as "going with the tide although my tide is different" and always looks toward the future (also characteristic of a veteran investment analyst).

When I asked him about the market, Irving replied, "doing what you're passionate about is much more important than worrying about what will happen in the market." Irving was not interested in going on about the subject; however, he has been quoted as saying that much of the unrest in the industry is due to "a bunch of gamblers going crazy on the floor of the exchange. Wall Street has always been a very poor judge of value."

At 106, Irving shows no signs of retiring, even though two of his three sons have already done so, one of them at literally half his age.

REACHING 100 & BEYOND! 106 YEARS

Lifestyle

General health	Irving's health has been excellent his entire life. He has never had a heart attack, stroke, cancer or any other serious illness.
Smoking	Smoked until he was in his 40s but quit cold turkey when one of his sons began emulating his habit.
Alcohol	An occasional social drink in his earlier years.

Nutrition	Irving "enjoyed home-cooked family dinners, chicken soup and a variety of foods." Although he didn't think much about a specific diet he always ate moderate portions and was always concerned about his weight. He was a bit overweight, but never obese.
Physical activity	Irving was very athletic in his earlier years, playing tennis, swimming, sailing and other sports. In recent years he's had no regimented exercise "except occasionally using light dumbbells" and while in his 90s he would sometimes walk the 20 blocks to work.
Current interests	Irving works every weekday in his office from 9 a.m. to 3 p.m. researching the market, and is a voracious reader of "purely non-fiction." He also enjoys reading *The Economist, Financial Times* and *The Wall Street Journal* daily.
Family	"I speak with my family every day." Irving has 3 sons (one who runs the company), 7 grandchildren and 11 great-grandchildren. He still lives in his apartment in Manhattan with the assistance of aides.

Family history

	AGE OF DEATH	CAUSE OF DEATH
Mother	80s	natural causes
Father	late 80s	natural causes
Sister	109	natural causes
Sister	102	natural causes
Brother	n/a	living, age 102

Factory Worker

Born: February 12, 1911, in Taunton, Massachusetts

Current Residence: Pearl River, New York

HELEN MULLIGAN

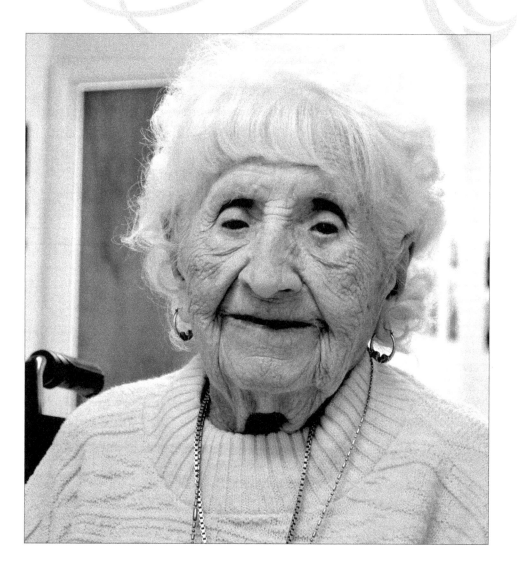

Words of Wisdom

101

"Take it easy, enjoy life, what will be will be. Sleep well, have a Bailey's Irish Cream before bed if you have a cold—you will wake up fine the next morning."

Although born in Massachusetts, Helen Mulligan's early years were spent under the guidance of her devoted grandmother in Poland. After Helen was born, her mother took her on a vacation to Poland. The grandparents decided they wanted her to stay with them, so her mother returned to Massachusetts to be with her husband. They moved to Connecticut, where they bore and raised the rest of their 5 children. Helen's father worked in a foundry and the mother was a housewife. When Helen was about 13 years old, her parents finally came back for her. Helen does not speak much about this time in her life, but one would imagine that it must have been quite difficult for her to understand why she was not raised with her siblings.

Balancing independence and uncertainty

Being quite independent at an early age, Helen went to work at 18. She heard about an opportunity to work as a nanny in New York City and decided to move there and live with some friends while she worked. However, her career was short-lived as just one year later she met her husband, Walter, left her job and had her first and only child two years later when she was 21.

Walter was rather successful working as a baker at a commercial bakery, even during the Great Depression. They did not have to worry like most, at least not at that time. However, after Helen and Walter were blissfully married for 18 years working and raising their daughter, tragedy came to their door. While Helen was just 37, her beloved husband was struck by bone cancer. According to Helen, "Walter died during the Great Blizzard of 1947, and was buried on the eve of our daughter's 16th birthday."

Thankfully, Helen's strong work ethic came in quite handy. With no education, her choices were limited, but she had to support her daughter. Helen got jobs working in various factories 40 hours a week. Fortunately for both mother and daughter, Helen met her second husband a few years later. His income gave them some relief but Helen still continued to keep her independence and worked diligently until she was 66. Her second husband passed away over 20 years ago of Alzheimer's at age 90.

Helen's daughter Mary says, "My mother was so inspiring as

"I was always very handy and active. In my 70s and onward, I was still pruning pine trees, mowing the lawn, cooking plentifully."

84

she never complained. She took life in stride and dealt with whatever obstacles came her way."

Still active in retirement

Although Helen rarely drinks, she insists that whenever she had a cold, a shot of Bailey's Irish Cream would "fix me by morning." And when asked which invention changed her life the most, she quickly responded, "the washing machine!"

"I was always very handy and active," explains Helen. "In my 70s and onward, I was still pruning pine trees, mowing the lawn, cooking plentifully and was constantly fixing things around the house. In my 80s, I became very involved with other seniors and participated in many activities at various senior centers. Initially, at 80, I felt too young to participate, but eventually I got involved with cooking and serving meals to residents."

Helen is still joyfully in service to her fellow seniors for over 20 years. She had slowed down due to a bad fall, which affected her mobility, however she still functions as the "money collector" at the senior center, at 101.

"My mother was so inspiring, she never complained. She took life in stride and dealt with whatever obstacles came her way."
— daughter Mary

"... at 80, I felt too young to participate."

Lifestyle

General health	Helen's health was generally good her entire life despite the diseases rampant in her family. She is on no medications currently and has never has been on medication on a regular basis. Beside some hearing and mobility loss, Helen is going strong.
Smoking	Smoked for 30 years, but quit 50 years ago. She lost two of her siblings who continued smoking, to lung cancer.
Alcohol	Rarely drank. But when she had a cold, she had some Bailey's Irish Cream and "licked it."
Nutrition	Besides eating oatmeal and bananas most mornings now, for most of her life, she ate mostly home-cooked Polish food such as pirogues, stuffed cabbage, polish sausage, and many vegetables such as spinach, cauliflower and salads with every meal. However, she ate very moderate amounts of food and was never obese, but at times "I had a few extra pounds." She only drank water and tea and about once per month went out to eat fast food.
Physical activity	Was always active doing her own cooking, house chores and gardening, even mowing her own lawn into her 70s and older. She also loved to dance the polka wherever possible.
Current interests	Volunteers at the senior center on a regular basis, cooks and enjoys watching the Yankees.

Family	Helen is very close with her daughter, with whom she lives, and has 3 grandchildren, 5 great-grandchildren and 8 great-great-grandchildren, with whom she is very close.

Family History

	AGE OF DEATH	CAUSE OF DEATH
Mother	89	pancreatic cancer
Father	60s	pneumonia
Sister	90	Parkinson's
Brother	n/a	alive at 85
Sister	74	lung cancer (smoker)
Brother	70	heart disease
Brother	70	heart disease
Brother	64	lung cancer (smoker)

It must have been quite difficult for her to understand why she was not raised with her siblings.

Real Estate Legend

Born: March 9, 1911, in Leslie, Arkansas

Current Residence: Dallas, Texas

EBBY HALLIDAY

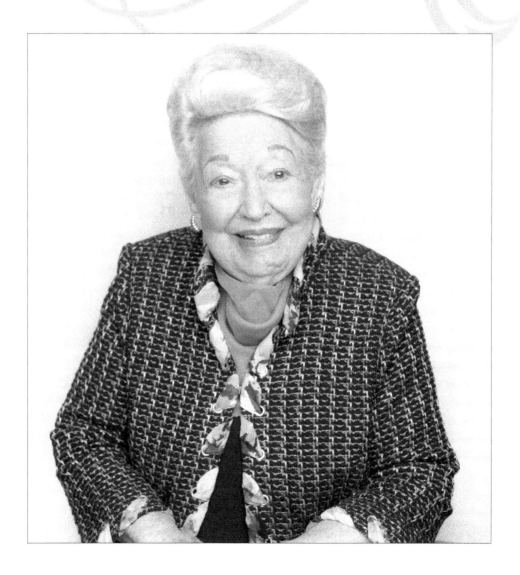

101 Words of Wisdom

"Don't smoke,
don't drink, and
don't retire!"

One of the first successful female entrepreneurs in Texas, and still, at 101, one of Dallas' leading businesswomen, Ebby Halliday built her real estate empire into an organization with over 1,500 sales associates and 30 state-of-the art offices. She's been invited to the White House to discuss economics and for Christmas dinner; has been on the board of too many associations to name; was chosen as Woman of the Year and Realtor of the Year on more than one occasion; and is one of only a few women ever to receive the coveted Horatio Alger award for her business achievements and philanthropy.

All of this achievement, yet from very humble beginnings. This is how her story unfolds...

A true entrepreneur since she was 11 years old

Vera Lucille Koch, now known by her preferred name, Ebby Halliday, was born in the small town of Leslie, Arkansas. When she was just three years old, her father, an engineer, was killed in a railroad accident at age 35. Her mother, brother and sister moved in with her grandparents, Reverend James Mabrey and his wife. Ebby's grandparents and mother instilled in Ebby the principles of worship, respect, gratitude and helping those less fortunate. This became Ebby's philosophy for her entire life.

Ebby's grandparents and mother instilled in Ebby the principles of worship, respect, gratitude and helping those less fortunate. This became Ebby's philosophy for her entire life.

A few years later, her mother, Lucille, married Fred Bigler, and they all moved to his 640-acre farm near Gypsum, Kansas. She said goodbye to the beautiful fruit orchards of the Arkansas Ozarks and hello to fields of wheat, corn and prairie dust. Life on this big, old farm was hard and dirty, but Ebby flourished. She would learn habits on that farm that would serve her well for a lifetime.

When Ebby was about eleven, wheat prices plummeted and her family fell on some very hard financial times. Her mom bore her fifth child, which made the strain even more difficult. Ebby recalls those days as some of the most challenging times in her life. But even at the age of eleven, Ebby found a way to help out her family. While flipping through a magazine, she noticed an advertisement for Cloverine salve. It seemed like a miracle ointment so she decided she was going to sell it for a few cents more than the purchase price. What made her think that her friends and neighbors would buy it from her versus the local drug store? Ebby would go door-to-door to

> A lady approached her and asked for help finding material for a quilt, explaining she made one for all of her grandchildren. In chatting together, Ebby learned that her seven sons all previously went to the same high school as Ebby was attending. One of her sons...
> Dwight D. Eisenhower.

each farm riding her pony, Old Deck. The youngster sold every tin she ordered as fast as the horse could trot.

Young Ebby also discovered that she could be more efficient distributing her sales at their one-room schoolhouse where children in all grades learned from the same teacher (envision *'Little House on the Prairie'*). Mothers would order the salve and Ebby would give the tins to the children to bring home... she was a natural entrepreneur.

Thinking out of the hat box

After graduating eigth grade, Ebby went on to high school with her sister Virginia forty-three miles away in Chapman, Kansas, as they both wanted a better education. They stayed with the postmaster and his wife. At 16, Ebby landed her first formal job at J.B. Case Department Store working part-time six days a week while in school to pay for her room and board. One summer while Ebby was working in the store, a lady approached her and asked for help finding material for a quilt, explaining she made one for each of her grandchildren. In chatting together, Ebby learned that the woman's seven sons all had gone to the same high school as Ebby was attending. One of her sons... Dwight D. Eisenhower.

91

Ebby wished to go to college but graduated from high school at the beginning of the Depression. As her family desperately needed her income, more schooling was out of the question. So Ebby continued to work. She was so successful in sales, that she was offered one promotion after another until she ended up in Dallas at W.A. Green Department Store selling hats.

An accidental real estate mogul

After working at W.A. Green for 6 years and growing their business, Ebby paid a visit to her doctor as she had a sore throat. She heard the doctor speaking about some investment he made in cotton futures and Ebby wanted in, so she invested $1,000 she had saved up. After 3 months, she parlayed her money into $12,000. Ebby quickly closed out and put the money toward a new business. After 17 years working in retail, Ebby opened her own hat boutique.

Ebby's small hat shop was doing very well. However, before long, the husband of one of her customers told her about his new home

He (the housing developer) said to Ebby, "If you can sell my wife these crazy hats, maybe you could sell my crazy houses."

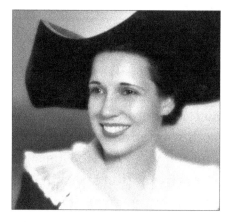

Photo courtesy of Ms Halliday

development consisting of 52 new cement-block insulated homes. He was having trouble selling them as they looked like prison blocks.

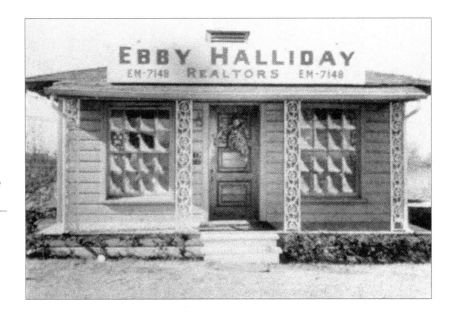

Ebby's first office. Photo courtesy of Ms Halliday

He said to Ebby, "If you can sell my wife these crazy hats, maybe you could sell my crazy houses." Ebby was very excited about this challenge and sold her hat business to her loyal designer, to take a stab at real estate. As quickly as she'd sold the Cloverine salve, she sold all 52 houses in the development.

The rest is history. Ebby went on to build the largest independently-owned residential real estate firm in Texas. A few years ago, it was on record that Ebby Halliday Realtors was the 10th largest realty business in the country.

Drive and creativity during difficult times

Ebby Halliday is a true inspiration to any businessperson going through a difficult time as she always found a way to make things work. Whether it was the Great Depression, WWII, or any other bleak economic era, Ebby always managed to do well in spite of it. In 1977, one of the hardest years economically, when inflation was high

One of her strongest passions was convincing women to believe that they can make a difference in the workplace, their communities and in government.

> "She considers it her obligation to give back to her community.

and mortgage rates were at 9% for a 30-year loan, Ebby's business had a record-breaking year. With a strong referral base, she received the business from the corporations who were relocating their executives. And with home prices going up, she also received larger commissions.

After almost seven decades in real estate, Ebby says she never forgets where she came from and how much she has learned from her experiences early on.

A true philanthropist who passionately served her community

Ebby was not just committed to growing her company, she was equally committed to enhancing her community, volunteering, raising funds for charities and local non-profit organizations. She participated in education programs and helped sponsor grants. In fact, she considered it her obligation to give back to her community. Ebby was involved in many organizations in real estate and philanthropy, and in most, she was eventually elected chairman or president.

> "Capitalism is when you have two cows: you sell one and buy a bull."

Ebby has also been called one of the most dynamic, convincing and inspiring speakers. She has traveled extensively around the world empowering women, students and even hard-nosed service managers at all-male oil refineries.

One of her strongest passions is convincing women to believe that they can make a difference in the workplace, their communities and in government. She knew from her own experience that women had the wherewithal and power within themselves to make that happen.

While she was developing Ebby Halliday Realtors into the success that it is, she met and married the love of her life, Maurice Acers. She was already 54 years old when they wed. Maurice worked for the FBI and thrilled Ebby with stories of his many operations. One Sunday, December 7, 1941, Maurice received a call from J. Edgar Hoover about some torpedoes that were dropped on Pearl Harbor in Hawaii. His role was to immediately round up the Japanese living in America that the FBI suspected might commit acts of sabotage, and relocate them to internment camps. The next day, President Roosevelt declared war on Japan.

After 27 years of a wonderful marriage, Maurice died of lung disease. In her biography, Ebby and Maurice's unique relationship was described as "a 27-year odyssey of work, personal growth, and volunteering."

> Ebby has been credited with single-handedly changing the face of real estate for women.

A woman way ahead of her time

Over 50 years ago, Ebby made it clear that she believed the government should stay out of the housing market, when at the time, the government was attempting to stabilize an overheated housing market by limiting the number of housing starts. Typical Ebby, she used this humorous example to make her point in one of her many speeches,

> *"Socialism is when you have two cows and you share the milk with everyone else. Communism is when you have two cows; the government takes the cows and gives you the milk. Fascism is when you have two cows; the government takes the cows and sells you the milk. Nazism is when you have two cows: the government takes the*

cows and shoots you. Capitalism is when you have two
cows: you sell one and buy a bull."

Still working today

Ebby has been credited with single-handedly changing the face of
real estate for women when she opened her first office nearly 70
years ago. She combined her business sense with feminine flair, and
made selling real estate a respected and fashionable profession for
women, which is still true today.

She continues to work in her realty company where she continues
as Chairman of the Board and attends many luncheons and dinners
of the many entities her company supports. On occasion, she even
finds time to delight audiences with her singing while playing the
ukulele!

After learning about Ebby's endless achievements and service
to others, I asked how she would want to be best remembered. She
simply stated, "as doing my best for family and friends."

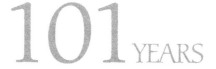

REACHING 100 & BEYOND!

Lifestyle

General health	Ebby's health was good most of her life and still is. However, around the age of 70, she had two non-malignant tumors removed—one in her head and one at the hairline.
Smoking	Never.
Alcohol	Never hard alcohol but an occasional wine.

Nutrition	"Having been raised on a farm, I ate nutritionally and was not overweight. I ate no junk food but lots of milk." Ebby takes iron and calcium supplements.
Physical activity	Physical fitness was very important to Ebby. She avidly played tennis, women's baseball and loved to ride horseback since she was a child.
Current interests	Ebby is very involved with her family, serves as Chairman of the Board at her large realty company and attends many luncheons and dinners of the many entities her company supports as well as political events.
Family	Ebby never had her own children, but Maurice had two daughters, seven grandchildren and ten great-grandchildren she speaks with often.

Family history

	AGE OF DEATH	CAUSE OF DEATH
Mother	70	kidney failure
Father	35	train accident
Brother	76	paranuclear palsy
Sister	70	morbid obesity
Brother	60	heart disease
Sister	40	unknown

WWII Veteran, Postal Worker, Eternal Bachelor (Well Almost!)
Born: March 24, 1912, in Rochester, New York
Current residence: Rochester, New York

GILBERT HERRICK

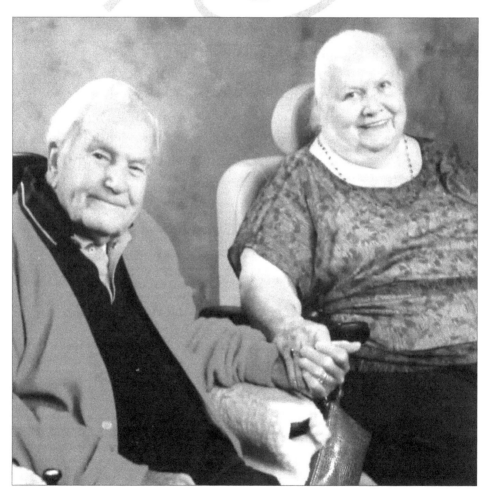

Gilbert and his new bride, Virginia.

Words of Wisdom

100

"Take one day at a time and go along with the tide."

Gilbert is a World War II veteran and a retired postal worker. He earned a Purple Heart Medal but was never able to fill his heart with the woman of his dreams until he turned 99!

It's never too late for love

Gilbert Herrick spent his entire life looking for Mrs. Right and, at the age of 99, he finally found her. "I never met the right woman until I met Virginia."

He had been living in a hospital/nursing home in Rochester, NY, for about 18 months with "nobody to talk to." Virginia Hartman-Herrick, 86, had been widowed for 25 years and moved to the same facility about 6 months after Gilbert did.

Gilbert has a passion for oil painting and was admiring some hand-painted china that was exhibited at the nursing home. He wanted to meet the artist, Virginia Hartman, and shortly thereafter, he was smitten. "I started visiting her every day. I thought she would kick me out." Well, she didn't. "We wanted to share a room, but you can't do that here unless you are married. So she asked me, and I said, yes."

Virginia's five children, grandchildren and great-grandchildren all helped prepare the wedding.

Overcoming life's challenges

Life indeed had its challenges for Gilbert. He is the oldest of seven siblings and has lost all but one. One of his brothers died at 7 years old due to a heart problem and they struggled through the Great Depression. "Food was really scarce."

Gilbert never finished high school but served in the US Army for 4 years during the war. "I was on three invasions—North

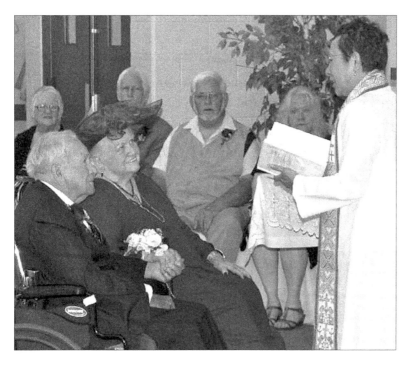

The Herricks' wedding ceremony.

Africa, Sicily and southern France and earned a Purple Heart." Following his service in the military, Gilbert worked for 30 years at the main post office until he retired in 1973 (a date which he remembers so vividly).

He had lived in the same home in Rochester for 97 years before moving to Monroe Community Hospital.

Golden and platinum years activities

When Gilbert was living at his home, he regularly gardened and took care of his yard. In his 80s, he started oil painting and traveled extensively around the world with his friends. One of his favorite trips to Hawaii was on his 80th birthday.

Gilbert hasn't been painting in the past few years, but is planning on painting once again with his new love, Virginia. As cute as can be, a source revealed that the two of them sometimes pass love notes back and forth, and then tear them up before anyone else sees what they have written.

Presently, Gilbert has a job. "I go to the greenhouse and unlock the door," he says. The MCH has a greenhouse where residents can indulge their horticultural interests. "They pay me $8 a month. I know it's not much for a married man."

Gilbert describes himself as "an ordinary person who is not a worrier."

He also travelled to Washington recently to visit the WWII Memorial courtesy of Honor Flight, an organization that flies veterans to the memorial for free. They thought Gilbert was too frail, but he was encouraged by his sweetheart to go, and he did.

Gilbert describes himself as "an ordinary person who is not a worrier." He lives his life taking one day at a time and just goes along with the flow. He and Virginia are living proof that love has no age and are committed to making the most out of the time they have together.

REACHING 100 & BEYOND! 100 YEARS

Lifestyle

General health	Heart disease runs rampant in the Herrick family. Although Gilbert has been generally healthy most of his life, he did survive a heart attack when he was 74.
Smoking	Never.
Alcohol	Never.
Nutrition	Gilbert ate a clean, wholesome diet most of his life. "I never ate fried foods and was never overweight."
Physical activity	Gilbert was physically active into his late 90s. Although he had no structured exercise, he was active as a postal worker into his 60s and would constantly garden and take care of the house and yard in his later years.
Current interests	His bride, Virginia and oil painting.
Family	Gilbert is recently married and lives with his wife. He was never married previously so he has no children.

Family history

	AGE OF DEATH	CAUSE OF DEATH
Mother	63	cancer
Father	52	heart attack
Sibling	7	heart attack
Sibling	65	heart attack
Sibling	75	heart attack
Sibling	87	cancer
Sibling	87	natural causes
Sibling	n/a	living, age 93

LILLIAN MODELL & GUSSIE LEVINE

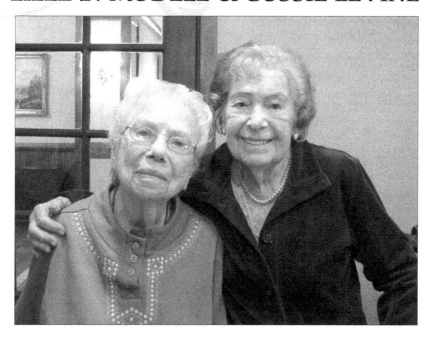

BEST FRIENDS AND
FELLOW CENTENARIANS

When I met fellow centenarians Gussie and Lillian at the beautiful FountainView Retirement Community in Monsey, NY, I immediately sensed that they had very different personalities and led very different lives. Regardless, they had been best friends for 12 years.

Gussie was very spiritual, thanking God for each day and taking life in stride. She said, "Each day is a gift from God and I see things happen when I talk to him." She had a good life, a very close family, good health for the most part.

Lillian, on the other hand, said, "I don't understand the significance of all the rituals as no one knows for sure of what, or who, God is." She, however, had a deep appreciation of our world, nature, human beings and the miracle of our existence. Unlike Gussie, she was a product of a very hard life, living in an orphanage for a good portion of her childhood, losing her father when she was only 4 years old, and dealing with 3 generations of family members with mental health issues.

> It has been said that kindred souls travel together.

Both Gussie and Lillian had impeccable cognitive ability. They recalled memories from 90 years ago as if they happened yesterday.

Sadly, both Gussie and Lillian passed away just months after this interview. It has been said that kindred souls travel together. They were born just 5 days apart and died within 3 months of each other, peacefully with their families by their side.

Teacher, Author of Children's Books

Born: July 20, 1910, in Manhattan, New York

Current residence: Monsey, New York

GUSSIE LEVINE

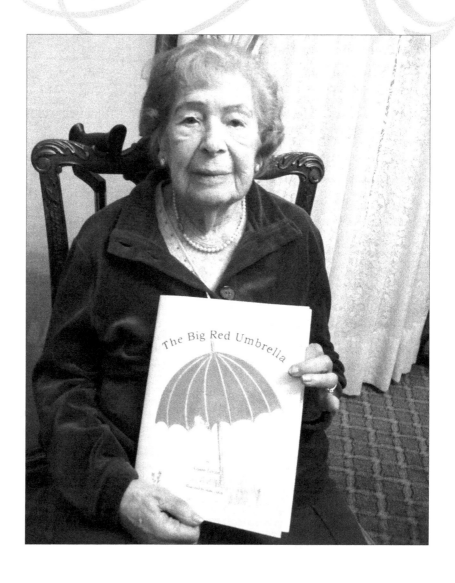

Words of Wisdom

100

"Don't fight the day, just let it be. Get up and be positive. Avoid any and all drama; I don't get involved with silly minutiae or difficult personalities; people respect me for that."

Born and bred in Manhattan, Gussie Levine attended Hunter College, graduating with a degree in Education. She married soon after, moved to Queens, "paid $36 a month for a one-bedroom apartment" and passionately taught for 24 years.

A loyal teacher and wife, then a new career at 96

A devoted wife, Gussie decided to retire early, in her 50s, after her husband had his first heart attack. She took care of him for many of her golden years. However, what was more inspiring and extraordinary about Gussie is what she achieved in her platinum years.

About 12 years ago, when Gussie was in her late 80s, she and her husband moved to the beautiful FountainView Retirement Community. Just 3 months later, her husband passed away. Instead of falling

> "I said to myself,
> 'I can write
> something better
> than that,'
> so I did."

into a state of loneliness or depression, Gussie picked up her life and became immersed in a series of adventures, activities and volunteerism. She went on a variety of trips, including a visit to the Challenger Center, not quite a week after celebrating her 100th birthday—where Gussie went on a simulated journey to the Moon! Ironically, it was on Gussie's 59th birthday in 1969 that Neil Armstrong took his famous trip to the Moon's surface—not simulated.

Gussie was a leader in her retirement community. She started a book club that met once a month and edited the weekly activity guide at the community center. She also held leadership positions in the Senior Club and Resident's Council.

Gussie was also a consummate volunteer. She was honored by RSVP (Retired and Senior Volunteer Program) as Volunteer of the Year in 2007 for her unconditional service for over 30 years. Her service included being a "foster grandparent" for pre-school children and a "phone friend" for kids in elementary school. She also volunteered at Nyack Hospital.

It was on one of her volunteer trips that she became inspired to write. "I was going with the seniors to read books to the children for the Head Start program. They picked up books from Woolworth's or some other store. I said to myself, 'I can write something better than that,' so I did."

At 96, Gussie Levine wrote and published her first children's book. Her daughter, Susan Lukin, created the illustrations. After she realized the book needed "something else," Gussie wrote a second one. And, when the second book needed something else, "I brought the characters from both books into my third book." Proceeds from sales of her books went to St. Jude's Children's Research Hospital.

Gussie's motto is to keep busy so she structures her activities every day. "Don't fight the day, just let it be. Get up and be positive."

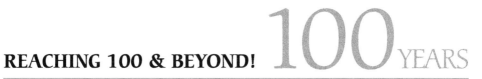

Lifestyle

General health	Gussie Levine was generally healthy into her platinum years.
Smoking	Never.
Alcohol	Never, except "an occasional Scotch on a Saturday with the Rabbi."
Nutrition	Always a "skinny kid", no eating out or take out, always home cooked, whole foods, loves vegetables, chicken and moderate treats.
Physical activity	Walked every morning 3 miles with her husband and goes on the treadmill 3 times per week even at 100
Current interests	"I always know what I am going to do each day." Book club, finances, editing weekly guide, volunteering, writing, trips, and other daily activities held at the center.
Family	Gussie is very close with her family who live nearby and speaks with them every day. She has 3 children, 3 grandchildren and 3 great-grandchildren.

Family history

	AGE OF DEATH	CAUSE OF DEATH
Mother	85	unknown
Father	85	unknown, died in sleep
Brother	95	natural causes
Brother	76	Parkinson's
Brother	14	accident, head injury
Brother	0	died at birth

Bookkeeper, Secretary, "Working Girl"

Born: July 15, 1910, in Manhattan, New York

Current residence: Monsey, New York

LILLIAN MODELL

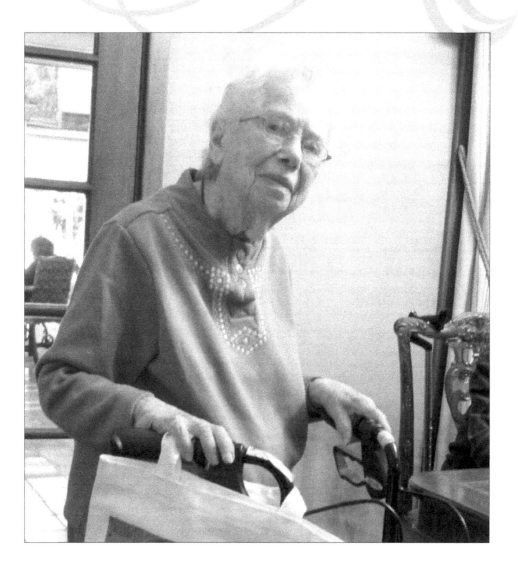

100 Words of Wisdom

"Keep busy!
Do things that you've
never done before."

At just 4 years old, Lillian had already dealt with great loss, the death of her father. Her mother told her that he went to visit Russia, was pulled into the Army, and was killed in service when he was in his 30s. Whether that story was true, we will never know. However, as there was "no welfare in those days," her mother had to work and had no one to care for young Lillian. Hence, Lillian had to be placed in foster care and then eventually ended up in an orphan asylum at the age of 7 with her little brother.

The first order of business when they arrived at the asylum: both children had to have their heads completely shaved to avoid lice.

Her extraordinary strength was challenged by turbulent times

Lillian remained there until she was 17 years old. Her mother came to visit her but Lillian always resented being there and told her so. Yet Lillian made the best of it and made a lot of friends there. She even maintained many of her friendships for several years and she said that her last friend from the orphanage just died recently. Lillian had outlived them all. Given her family situation, friends were always of utmost importance to her.

Soon after she was "liberated" from the orphanage, Lillian became a self-proclaimed "working girl." She got her first job as a bookkeeper and then became a school secretary for several years. However, just a few years later, Lillian once again was handed an enormous challenge. She was 22 years old when she met her future husband, Mac, but was completely unaware that he had a family history of mental illness. After only 3 months of marriage, Mac started to exhibit symptoms of mental illness. "For years, I was living on the edge wondering when he was going to break down again." Her marriage was indeed very turbulent and in addition to dealing with this challenge, Lillian took her mother in—yes, the very person who placed her in the orphanage as a young child—to live with them, as the mother could not afford to be on her own.

Six years later, Lillian

> "For years, I was living on the edge, wondering when he was going to break down again."

> Lillian took her mother in— yes, the very person who placed her in the orphanage.

gave birth to her first daughter who inherited the mental illness running in her husband's family. To make matters worse, her daughter's two children inherited the disease as well. Lillian somehow managed to stop working for a while so that she could be around for her children as her parents had not been there for her. Once the children reached middle school, Lillian went back to work full-time, while taking care of her husband and mother. Lillian was married for 40 years. Fortunately, her second daughter, Cora, did not develop any mental issues and, as Lillian says, truly became her savior. "She is my life support, she does everything for me."

> *Friends and family would constantly ask her for favors, and she would gladly oblige.*

> *"I started doing things that I've never done before."*

"I let a lot pass, but I also kept a lot in. I learned how to cope well given what I had to go through in life." According to her daughter, Lillian didn't focus much on her own difficulties; she focused more on helping others. Her daughter said, "We had an open door policy. She was probably the busiest person out of all of her friends and family, but they would constantly come by our house and ask her for favors, and she would gladly oblige."

Still a busy, productive woman in her later years

"After retiring, I immediately became bored, so I volunteered." Lillian volunteered in two nursing homes for 19 years. She also took a job one day a week doing bookkeeping well into her 80s. She was 88 when she came to FountainView's assisted living which was a whole new world for her. "I started doing things that I've never done before." She became the editor of their newsletter, secretary of the senior club and facilitator of the knitting group. She even had the opportunity to sell her sweaters. "Lillian also loves to paint," best friend Gussie Levine chimed in, "and she's very good at it." Lillian attended night classes in painting as a young adult and painted on and off her whole life. She was also the oldest person ever to visit the Challenger Center for Space Science Education to simulate a journey to the moon.

Lillian is an example of a woman who is quite extraordinary, not because of an illustrious career or academia, but due to her extraordinary strength, generosity and tenacity despite the most difficult of times.

REACHING 100 & BEYOND! 100 YEARS

Lifestyle

General health	Lillian was in good health until she developed diabetes later in life. However, through her diet, she was able to manage it well.
Smoking	Never.
Alcohol	No, just an occasional social drink.
Nutrition	Lillian always ate well and kept her weight down. She was of average weight throughout her life and "was a skinny kid." She cooked most of the time, as they could not afford to eat out. "We didn't know from ordering a pizza. I was a very careful shopper and cook. I still make my own breakfast and lunch." She likes most foods and made sure her diet was balanced. She also took multivitamins regularly.

Physical activity	She never drove so she walked everywhere and up and down several flights of stairs to and from her apartment.
Current interests	Knitting, painting, editing weekly newspaper at the senior center, various field trips and other activities held at the center.
Family	Lillian has 2 daughters, one she sees very frequently, 4 grandchildren and 2 great-grandchildren who come to visit her.

Family history

	AGE OF DEATH	CAUSE OF DEATH
Mother	76	stroke from diabetes and high blood pressure
Father	30s	died in Russian Army
Brother	88	prostate cancer

Lillian ended up in an orphan asylum at the age of 7 with her little brother.

Seamstress

Born: May 12, 1911, in Italy

Current residence: Nanuet, New York

JENNIE CASCONE

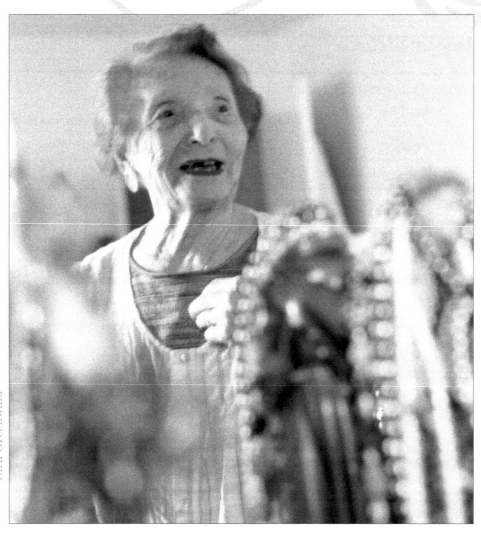

Tara Greenwald

Words of Wisdom

100

"Be good, don't complain, just get up and do. Keep on working, keep on going, and have a good time."

Although Jennie is quite petite, her exuberance makes her quite a powerhouse. Entertaining and wise, it is no wonder why I wanted to adopt her as the great-great-grandmother I never had. Her essence just radiated joy and it was rather contagious. Jennie made me believe that no matter what challenges you face, and no matter how old you become, you can still appreciate life, be light and warm, and enjoy your life.

Hard work and hard times

At the young age of 9, Jennie and her family left Italy and immigrated to the United States. Just 9 years later, Jennie got married and moved to the big city—into Manhattan—with her husband.

At 100 years old, Jennie vividly remembers her exact address,

294 Cherry Street. She also remembers when her husband lost his job during the Great Depression and found another job making $15 every other week. Although it was difficult, Jennie says modestly, "Everything was so much cheaper in those days anyway, it wasn't so bad."

After World War II, Jennie went to work as a seamstress in the Garment District for a family-run business for over 36 years. She worked hard but it was a labor of love.

All was going well until tragedy struck. Jennie lost both her mother and her father from illness just 5 months apart. Her mother was only 57 and her father was 60 when they died. Still grieving for her beloved parents, Jennie subsequently contracted hepatitis from a blood transfusion. She spent 79 days in the hospital.

Not one to stand idle, Jennie went right back to work as soon as she was released. She loved what she did and whom she worked for. "I worked for a Jewish family so I learned to speak Yiddish. I was the Yiddish shiksah!" In addition to Yiddish and English, Jennie also speaks Italian and Polish.

"I learned to speak Yiddish. I was the Yiddish shiksah!"

A true giver who stays busy

After retiring at age 62, Jennie devoted herself to taking care of her husband, who was 10 years her senior and was suffering from a series of strokes. Her husband passed away when Jennie was 79.

Jennie has kept busy doing what she does best—giving, sharing and spreading joy to those around her. She joined the Meals on Wheels Senior Center and has been volunteering there for almost 20 years helping out in the kitchen and enjoying the fellowship and activities. She was participating every day for many years and is still participating three days per week.

In addition to her visits to the senior center, Jennie does her own cooking and cleaning and enjoys knitting in her warm, lovely home

Jennie joyfully danced around her kitchen floor as she sang her mantra, "Que sera, sera, whatever will be, will be..."

where she lives with her daughter, Jean, her only child, who is 80 years old. Jennie likes to wake up early in the morning and walk around for exercise, then she watches some television before heading to the center. She even went to Atlantic City within the past year and donated her winnings to the senior center.

During our interview, Jennie joyfully danced around her kitchen floor as she sang her mantra, *"Que sera, sera, whatever will be, will be... I have restless leg syndrome, but I can still dance!"* The song reflects her wonderful mental outlook of living each day to the fullest and not sweating the small stuff. What an inspiration!

When Jennie turned 100, the senior center and her family acknowledged her wonderful nature, generosity and spirit by throwing her two tremendous parties. Jennie said she had the time of her life.

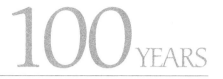
Lifestyle

General health	About 40 years ago, Jennie had a severe ulcer and developed hepatitis from a blood transfusion. Besides that, she never had a health problem.
Smoking	Never.
Alcohol	Never.
Nutrition	Most everything was homemade. "My family always ate together, always vegetables on our plate." Per her daughter, Jennie lived on a very healthy Mediterranean diet,which she learned from her Italian heritage. She typically ate greens, fruits, beans and olive oil and was never overweight. Now she eats sparsely and enjoys eggs and fruit cups. Jennie quips, "I better go with a full stomach when I die."
Physical activity	Danced regularly and was "always active."
Current interests	Volunteering at the senior center, involved in various activities including helping out in the center's kitchen, still cooks and cleans house.
Family	Lives with her daughter with whom she has a wonderful relationship. Her twin sister lives in upstate New York. Jennie has 3 grandchildren and 1 great-grandchild.

Family history

	AGE OF DEATH	CAUSE OF DEATH
Mother	57	diabetes and high blood pressurre led to stroke
Father	60	asthma
Sister (twin)	still living	100 years old
Brother	75	cancer
Brother	67	diabetes and gangrene
Brother	47	heart attack
Brother	unknown	cancer

Her essence just radiated joy and I found it was rather contagious.

Attorney, Philanthropist

Born in 1912 (exact month unknown) in Ukraine

Current residence: Philadelphia, Pennsylvania

MURRAY H. SHUSTERMAN

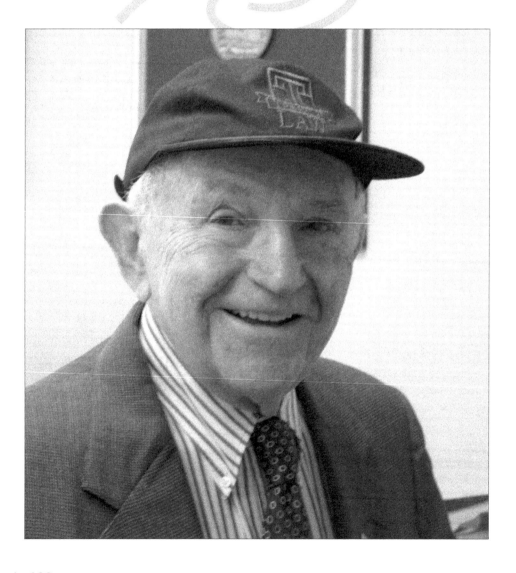

Words of Wisdom

100

"Get involved. You'll find pleasure and sometimes disappointment but there is a sense of achievement if you participate in a successful undertaking, whether it is organizational or professional. Work hard, it will pay off."

As I waited in the palatial lobby on the floor housing Mr. Murray Shusterman's office, out comes an incredibly youthful centenarian walking over to greet me. As we were passing the receptionist on the way to his office, Murray leans over her desk and whispers loudly, "This young lady came here from New York to convince me to run the marathon."

A blend of brilliance, generosity, wit and charm

This line was a prelude to Murray's playful wit and charm. Murray Shusterman is as sharp as a tack with a remarkable memory, lives completely independently and is still a practicing attorney, a senior partner in a large law firm for over 47 years. I felt as if I were speaking with someone a decade or two older than myself, certainly not five.

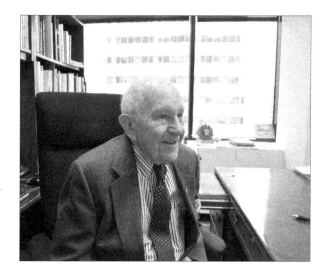

Murray, a proud Temple U Law School alumni, in his office.

When I had initially called to schedule a time with Murray for this interview, I was concerned that it might cut into his lunch. When I expressed my concern, Murray responded, "I've been fasting on Yom Kippur for 90 years, so I think I can hold out awhile for lunch."

A passion for the law

Murray was born in a small village in the Ukraine and came to America when he was 7 years old. He doesn't know his exact birthday, as there were no records where he had lived. "My mother told me she thought my birthday was in August, but when I got older and realized that I couldn't celebrate an August birthday in school, I chose my own date in the week after Labor Day so I can have a party too."

Murray lived in Philadelphia most of his life. He attended Temple University Law School and then went on to University of Pennsylvania for his Masters in Political Science and his "PhDabd" (PhD All But the Dissertation). He never found time to finish his dissertation once his first son was born. First he worked individually as a lawyer and then as a partner

He jokes, "I've been here over 47 years, although no one asks me to be their Executor or Trustee (for obvious reasons)."

124

at Fox and Rothschild where he is still practicing. He jokes, "I've been there over 47 years, although no one asks me to be there Executor or Trustee—for obvious reasons."

"I remember seeing men in suits in the streets selling apples."

"Even when I was in grade school, I knew I wanted to be a lawyer," says Murray. When he started his practice, it was at the end of the Great Depression when unemployment reached new levels. "I had worked to earn my tuition and remember seeing men in suits in the streets selling apples. During the Great Depression, my father was in the embroidery business and had such strong ethics he just couldn't lay off any employees, so my wife, Judith, and I moved in with my parents after we married to help pay the rent. When the war came and my father had the machinery to make epaulettes and so on, my parents did so well that they became very affluent. Only in America!"

Although Murray is greatly passionate about the law and serving justice, he admits that he has lost plenty of sleep over the suffering he had witnessed from victims, their families and even the perpetrators' families.

A supporter of civil liberties and Temple University

A former senior vice president of B'nai B'rith International and chairman of the B'nai B'rith Klutznick Museum, Murray now serves as chairman of the International

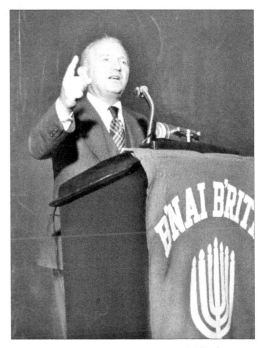

125

Advisory Council, as a member of the International Board of Governors and as president of the B'nai B'rith World Center in Jerusalem. B'nai B'rith is the oldest Jewish community service organization in the world.

On his desk sit photos of Murray welcoming presidents Reagan, Carter and Bush Sr. to various conventions. Murray also sits on the Board of Trustees of Ben Gurion University and has been to Israel at least 30 times for meetings.

Although very active in the Jewish community, interestingly enough Murray is not very religious. He supports Jewish rights and

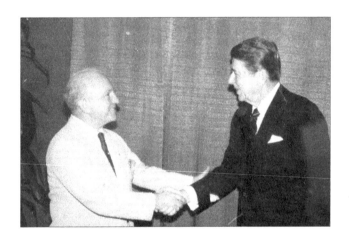

Murray welcoming President Reagan to a B'nai B'rith Convention. Photo courtesy of Mr. Shusterman

culture, observes the holidays, but still grapples with how a "God can permit thousands of people to die in a tsunami or millions to perish in the Holocaust."

Murray is also a devoted and generous alumnus and supporter of Temple University and its law school. As a senior adjunct professor, he taught corporate and real estate law for more than 30 years. He is president of the Law Foundation, which he helped found; a former president of the Temple Law Alumni; and an Honorary Life Trustee of the university. In 1981, he established the Murray H. Shusterman Fellowship/Scholarship, a major fund that supports the exchange of Temple and Israeli law students, faculty and scholars.

As a result of his generosity, Shusterman Hall sits proudly at Temple University Law School, serving as a multi-functional, state-of-the-art educational and meeting facility.

Reaching his platinum years

Murray was married in 1940 to his beloved Judith, a union that lasted for 64 years. "She was a brilliant woman." Judith passed away "exactly 6 years and 12 days ago." They had 3 sons, 10 grand-children and 3 great-grandchildren. "I have very close relationships with my children," Murray said as he proudly rattled off some of their many achieve-ments. "My kids are smart, they took after their mother."

> "I wanted a place on the golf course, Judith wanted a place on the ocean, so we compromised and bought a place on the ocean."

In his early 80s, Murray and Judith purchased a second home on the ocean in Florida and were very active there. Murry quips, "I wanted a place on the golf course, Judith wanted a place on the ocean, so we compromised and bought a place on the ocean." Murray loved to play golf and joined a walking club.

> "One of the saddest parts of my life today, is that every one of my friends is dead, every one!"

Coping with loss

Murray was generally healthy most of his life except for a bypass about 6 years ago. When I asked him if he found it challenging at times being this old, he replied, "One of the saddest parts of my life today is that every one of my friends is dead, every one!" He explained how most people in his generation didn't live much past 60.

How does he cope with losing all of his peers? "I get along with young people. I consider myself a friendly person with a sense of humor. I don't hate strongly, but dislike certain people and certain things annoy me, but I am apt to forgive." He adds mischievously, "I forgive differently than a woman though, who is willing to forgive as well, but will never forget what she forgave."

REACHING 100 & BEYOND! 100 YEARS

Lifestyle

General health	Murry was generally healthy his whole life.
Smoking	Murray was smoking a half pack a day plus a pipe regularly, but stopped over 50 years ago when "my younger son said that he heard that you can die from it." He made a pact with his sons that he would stop if they would swear (raising right hand and all) never to start. They proceeded to break apart his Camel cigarettes and he never smoked again.
Alcohol	Only a drink or two at occasional parties.
Nutrition	Murray has never been overweight and for most of his life has enjoyed home-cooked meals. His mother always prepared fresh vegetables and meats and his wife introduced him to many new, wholesome foods. He is now a self-proclaimed "warmer-upper", buying freshly prepared soups, vegetables, chicken and leftovers from family dinners. He also eats at his country club and dines out elsewhere as well. He regularly takes vitamins C and D.

Physical activity	Member of his walking club in Florida. "You have the younger walkers (guys in their 80s), then you have us AKs—*alda kackers*—Yiddish for older guys." He's always been active except for the past year, but he still plays golf.
Current interests	Until his wife passed, he traveled with her all over the world. Besides working as an attorney and his involvement in philanthropic ventures, he still walks, plays golf, and plays bridge.
Family	Has very close relationships with his 3 sons, 10 grandchildren and 3 great-grandchildren.

Family history

	AGE OF DEATH	CAUSE OF DEATH
Mother	90s	complications from a fall
Father	72	stomach cancer, very heavy smoker
Sister	late 80s	unknown
Sister	late 80s	unknown
Brother	30s	unknown disease

Murry is a blend of brilliance, generosity, wit and charm.

Book Binder, Adventurer
Born: July 26, 1908, in Bronx, New York
Current residence: New City, New York

ANNE LOMEDICO

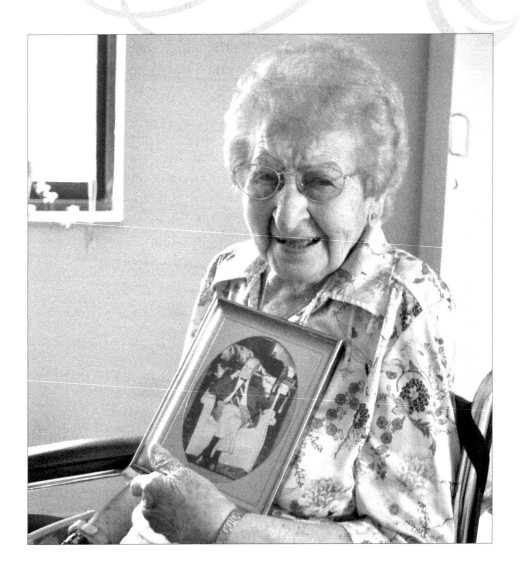

Words of Wisdom

104

"I had a wonderful marriage for 61 years, was active and danced my whole life, but I believe my life is in God's hands."

Strong, loyal and hardworking, Anne LoMedico has been "Anne the Adventurer" from pre-teen to "platinum." Her adventurous personality came into play at the age of 14 when she left school to look for a job. The family was in desperate need of money and Anne was determined to help them. Potential employers turned Anne away time and time again even though she was using her older sister's birth certificate.

The authorities eventually caught her. Anne went to court and after relentlessly pleading with the judge, was given an exemption from school in order to look for a job. The judge even helped her find one.

Anne's first job was working at a factory making $7 per week. Although she received a promotion to $9 per week, Anne decided to leave and begin her new vocation at Charles H. Bohn & Co., a Manhattan bookbindery where she worked loyally for 50 years. She started as a machine operator and worked her way up to supervisor in a short time. She did everything from "putting the covers on the books to desk work." Anne became a union delegate and at one time was awarded a gold pin by the Bookbinders Union due to her initiative and hard work.

Anne married her beloved Carmelo about five years after she started working and raised two children. This was all during the Great Depression. Anne does not like to talk about the Great Depression, as it was an extremely difficult time for them. There was so little food and work (Carmelo was in construction) but she and her husband refused to go on welfare.

The sudden death of her son of a heart attack at age 46, which Anne said was the most challenging time of her life, was the pivotal moment that solidified her decision to retire at age 67.

Since the age of 80, "Anne has made almost 2 dozen trips around the world, has rode on a camel, in a hot air balloon, on a mechanical bull, in a helicopter and has walked on a glacier. If it was there to do, she did it."
– Marie, Anne's daughter

If it was there to do it, she did it

In 1988, Anne and Carmelo decided to move from the city to suburban Rockland County, New York to be near their daughter. A few years later, Carmelo passed away. Although she lost the love of her life, Anne still kept on living and, boy, did she know how to live. According to her daughter, since then, in her 80s, "Anne has made almost two dozen trips around the world, has rode on a camel, in a hot air balloon, on a mechanical bull, in a helicopter and has walked on a glacier. If it was there to do, she did it."

Anne also loved to sing and dance. When I asked her what she thought had defined her, she responded, "being in a play in my 80s for 12 years with the Clarkstown Seniors."

Until very recently, Anne kept busy splitting her time between the Nyack Senior Center and Congers Senior Club 6 days a week participating in various activities and fundraisers. I was apprised by one of the administrators that when she was 99 she raised the most money for their annual Walkathon in which she too participated. She's also helped many women in her community who have recently been widowed to keep active and get back into life.

In her late 90s, she boldly asked one of the centers to add another exercise class to their schedule. And, just like she won over the judge when she was 14 years old, she won these administrators over too.

Anne attributes her extreme longevity to her long, happy marriage, eating right, staying active, never smoking and her strong faith.

Anne the Matriarch

Anne grew up with nine siblings in the Bronx borough of New York City and is the only one still living. Some of her siblings reached their 90s, but she did experience great tragedy amongst them at a young age. Two of her siblings succumbed to heart disease and leukemia in their 40s. Her older brother, who was gassed during WWI when she was a child, became very sick soon after and died years later at 57 from the effects of the poison gas.

Although various diseases took the lives of her family members, Anne never had any serious illness in her life. However, she has had a surgery here and there for structural issues. Spinal stenosis

"Anne is a very strong, confident woman who lives day to day."

was affecting the mobility in her arms in her 90s and she insisted on having surgery to repair it, despite the risk. At 101, her spine affected her ability to walk (which is why now she is in a wheelchair) and she insisted on having surgery again. This time, she was refused. Her motto was: "If it could be fixed, fix it!" as she never wanted to live in pain nor with restrictions. The family often referred to her as the 'bionic woman.'

Anne had 2 children, and currently has 7 grandchildren, 19 great-grandchildren and 10 great-great-grandchildren. Her husband passed away after 61 "wonderful" years of marriage. Anne had been living with her daughter, Marie, but now lives at a rehabilitation center since she has had issues with her legs.

Although her extended family is spread out all over geographically, on her 100th birthday a few years back, 125 of them came together to celebrate. She is also very close with the other club members who had thrown her a surprise party as well.

As described by her family, "Anne is a very strong, confident woman who lives day to day." We could all take note of that.

REACHING 100 & BEYOND! 104 YEARS

Lifestyle

General health	Although heart disease was prevalent in her large family, Anne never had any disease during her life.
Smoking	Never.

134

Alcohol	Only on special occasions.
Nutrition	Regularly cooked "moderate portions of meat and pasta with lentils, beans, vegetables, always with a salad." Anne was never overweight.
Physical activity	Danced and exercised regularly until present. Walked a few miles to work every day.
Current interests	Involved with many activities at the senior center including exercise, bingo, as well as her many adventures as described above. Travelled worldwide in her 80s and beyond.
Family	Only survivor of 10 siblings. Two children, seven grandchildren, 19 great-grandchildren and 10 great-great-grandchildren. Lived with her daughter until one year ago. Married 61 years, widowed over 20 years.

Family history

	AGE OF DEATH	CAUSE OF DEATH
Mother	61	heart attack
Father	90	natural causes
Sister	90s	natural causes
Sister	90s	natural causes
Brother	80s	lung cancer (smoker)
Sister	80s	muscular sclerosis
Brother	80s	Alzheimer's
Sister	70s	stroke
Brother	57	gassed in WWI
Sister	46	leukemia
Brother	40s	heart attack

Dancer

Born: November 1, 1912, in Brooklyn, New York

Current residence: Boca Raton, Florida

ANNE LAMONT

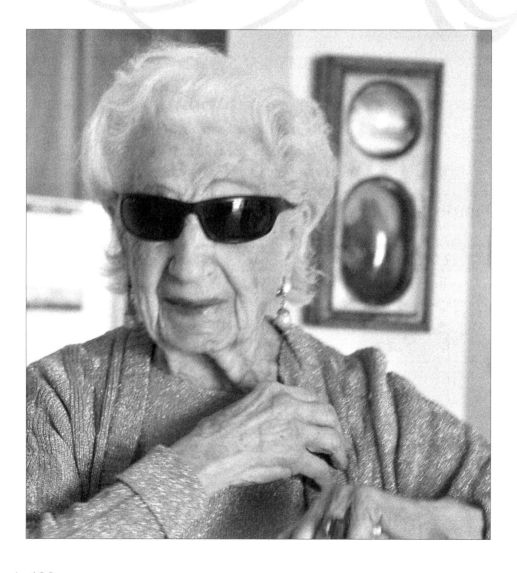

Words of Wisdom

100

*"Think positively and
enjoy your children,
enjoy your life."*

Anne Lamont was the sixth of nine siblings and grew up
very poor. In those days, it was typical that the children
pitched in to help support the family, so Anne left high
school to find a job. She managed to land work at various shoe companies, which wasn't easy during the Great Depression. However,
Anne worked hard and played hard.

In the face of challenge, just dance

Anne loved to dance and despite her circumstances would religiously
venture out to dance with her friends every weekend. Her favorite
dance was the "Peabody", a peculiar quickstep type dance where
the partner is held way out to the right, rather than in front. And
Anne was rather good at it. So good, in fact, that she won several

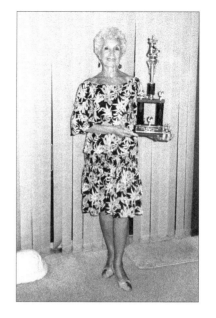

Anne Lamont, stunning at 85 years old, receiving an award for "Best Peabody" at the Gold Coast Ballroom. Photo courtesy of Anne Lamont

awards for the Peabody, her last one she received at 85 years old at the Gold Coast Ballroom in Florida. Her daughter said that people would stand in awe of her mother and her various dance partners as they swept the dance floor. And, at 100, Anne is still dancing.

> "I slept with a statue of St. Jude and would take it with me all day, every day. I would pray to him to help me get through a lot of things. He was my patron saint."

Anne met her husband in the Catskill Mountains of New York while she was, yes, dancing, and they fell in love. They got married when she was 27 and had two children. Although she had a wonderful marriage for 38 years, it was often quite challenging, as her husband was manic-depressive. She supported her husband during his shock treatments and many difficult episodes, but through all of it, they both found time to dance. "We would go to Roseland in Manhattan on a regular basis."

Besides dancing, Anne had another method of dealing with life's challenges: her strong faith. "I slept with a statue of St. Jude and would take it with me all day, every day. I would pray to him to help me get through a lot of things. He was my patron saint."

While raising her children, Anne worked several part-time jobs including one at her children's school cafeteria, at a bakery and even a candy factory. At the candy factory, she would get paid for every box she filled. "Every candy fit into the box until the last one. Once I put the last one in, all of the candies would pop out." Her daughter, Judy, who would often help her mother at the factory after school with her sister, described it like an episode of the comedy show *I Love Lucy*.

> *She confidently wore a leotard, fishnet stockings and black stilettos. Her daughter and granddaughter were aghast.*

Nine lives and lots of nerve

At 65, after her husband passed away, Anne moved to Florida by herself and bought a small mobile home. She then moved to an independent living facility where she got involved in various club activities, including dancing and acting.

At 80, Anne played a barroom hooker in one of the community plays. She confidently wore a leotard, fishnet stockings and black stilettos. Her daughter and granddaughter were aghast.

Daughter, granddaughter and great-grandchildren visit Anne frequently at her Florida home.

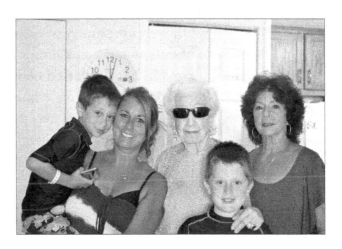

In her later years, you could say that Anne had "nine lives." When she was 80, she beat breast cancer. At 82, she had a quadruple bypass. At 87, she had shingles and Bell's palsy, which caused her eye to close due to nerve damage in her face. Although she claims that the Bell's palsy greatly affected her spirit as it altered her physical appearance, she still seemed quite audacious to me as she struck Madonna-like dance poses while she was being photographed.

At 93, Anne fell down a flight of stairs, headfirst, but miraculously broke nothing. Her daughter attributes her physical resilience and agility to her inveterate dancing throughout her life.

Anne is the lone survivor of a family of 9 siblings.

REACHING 100 & BEYOND! 100 YEARS

Lifestyle

General health	Before she reached her 80s, Anne was in very good health.
Smoking	Yes, but she quit while in her 20s.
Alcohol	Rarely, except for occasional wine homemade by her grandfather.
Nutrition	Anne benefitted from a fresh Mediterranean diet as her family was born in Italy. Her family would pick dandelion weeds from the lots in Brooklyn and boil them. Her father made his own olive oil and her grandfather his own wine. She ate everything in moderation and was never overweight.
Physical activity	Anne always kept herself trim by dancing and walking regularly.

Current Interests	Until her recent bout with severe dizziness from Bell's palsy, Anne regularly participated in the daily and evening activities at her senior community complex.
Family	Anne sees her daughter, granddaughter and great-grandchildren who reside nearby quite frequently. She has 2 daughters, 4 grandchildren, and 4 great-grandchildren.

Family history

	AGE OF DEATH	CAUSE OF DEATH
Father	95	natural causes
Mother	75	stroke
Sister	99	natural causes
Brother	90s	natural causes
Brother	90s	natural causes
Brother	90s	natural causes
Sister	82	Alzheimer's
Brother	60s	heart attack
Brother	60s	heart attack
Brother	2	unknown

Anne would dance with her friends every weekend.

Traveling Salesman, Family Man

Born: August 19, 1911, in East New York

Current residence: Monsey, New York

MORRIS LENSKY

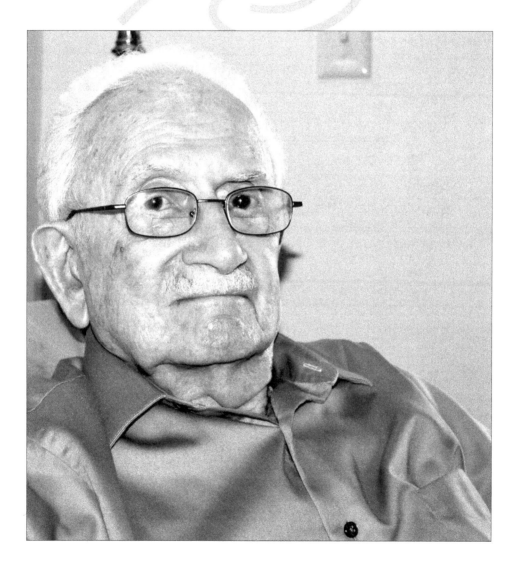

Words of Wisdom

101

"You have to be lucky, but I made the best of things when bad things happened. I also ate prunes every single day."

I met with Morris ("Murray") Lensky, his daughter Lorrie, and his granddaughter Alisa, in his residence at FountainView, a beautiful independent retirement community in Monsey, New York. He was a friendly, sweet and genuine man. What I found so extraordinary about Murray was his incredible desire for independence, even at 100, and his undying love and loyalty toward his family. He was a simple man who worked hard his whole life, but, according to his family, no matter what his circumstances, he never ever complained. What a beautiful role model for his family and for us all.

A harrowing experience en route to America

Murray began the interview with the harrowing story of how he came into this world.

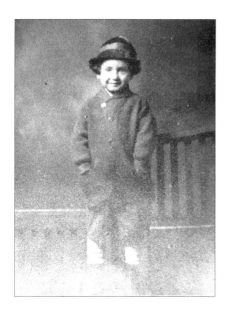

Young Murray. Courtesy of Murray Lensky

"The family all lived in Romania. My father wanted a better life for us so he sent my mother, pregnant with me, on a boat to America. He would meet us there as soon as he was able. What he didn't expect was the language barrier would pose a real problem. Authorities suspected that I was an illegitimate baby as my mother was alone, and wanted to take me away from her. As my mother only spoke Yiddish, she was unable to explain the situation. Fortunately, when we got to New York City, she found a doctor who understood Yiddish and was able to read a letter from my father. I was saved."

Although it was a rough start for his family, Murray was very proud of his father who managed to raise enough money for himself and his mother's entire family to come to the USA from Romania.

The traveling salesman

Murray grew up in the Bronx, graduated from City College and wanted more than anything to be a dentist. However, things didn't go as planned. Not long before his graduation, Murray's father lost all of the family's money when Wall Street collapsed in the 1929 stock market crash. Dad couldn't afford to send him to school.

Realizing he couldn't follow that dream due to circumstances, Murray pressed on and explored other ventures. He decided to become a traveling salesman, selling magazines and "other items you would find in the department stores." He adds, "In those days there were no credit cards, people would pay me in increments, typically $5 per week. I would buy the items wholesale on the lower east side and sell them at a profit. Sometimes, I would actually bring customers downtown to look at items or bring jewelry to them. They couldn't buy online in those days."

Murray's hard work paid off, as he became a very successful man.

In 1941, he met Pearl, the love of his life whom he proposed to on their second date, and quickly started a family.

A loyal husband through and through

After 40 years of working and raising two children, Murray and Pearl retired to sunny Florida and enjoyed it for over 20 years. They walked together every day and Murray played golf. They also enjoyed an active social life.

Unfortunately, this blissful life would be cut short when Pearl contracted Alzheimer's, the same disease that took Murray's mother's life. His children and grandchildren attest that in all the years Murray took care of Pearl, he was never stressed and never complained. He just dealt with it, always stayed calm and did what he needed to do. And he insisted on caring for Pearl all on his own.

This trait of loving loyalty came from his mother. What stood out most in their family was the constant love surrounding it. According to his daughter, "Dad's mother was the most loving, caring, compassionate woman who lived for her children." Murray, in turn, lived for his children and loved and supported his wife until the very end.

This trait of loving loyalty came from his mother.

145

Eventually Murray conceded and moved back to New York to accept some help from the family. After 63 years of marriage, Pearl passed away.

Independent yet close with family

At 101, Murray still lives independently in a retirement facility that exudes old world charm. He still loves to exercise, play cards weekly, goes to shows regularly, and is a voracious reader. Murray loves to learn. He remains very close with his loving family and cherishes his time with them. And he still never complains.

REACHING 100 & BEYOND! 101 YEARS

Lifestyle

General health	Murray's general health was always excellent. He has been on no medication except for blood pressure treatment to prevent it from falling to low.
Smoking	"Tried it once in college and never since."
Alcohol	Only Maneshewitz wine on the holidays.
Nutrition	Murray's mother and wife were both "excellent cooks who cooked healthy" according to his daughter and granddaughter. He was and is a very moderate eater, likes fish and eats meat occasionally. Although now he admits he has a doughnut every morning for breakfast, he doesn't eat much and was always trim. He eats prunes, takes a multivitamin and calcium daily.

Physical activity	Murray is still on the stationary bicycle 2 to 3 times per week. He used to walk everyday with his wife and later with his girlfriend, Sally, and was an avid golfer.
Current interests	Murray loves to learn. He reads constantly *Readers Digest, Smithsonian* and, for pure enjoyment, detective stories. He plays cards weekly and likes to go to the shows at the FountainView monthly.
Family	One daughter who he sees regularly. One son who lives in California but speaks with him daily, four grandchildren and six great-grandchildren. He also sees his daughter's family on a regular basis.

Family history

	AGE OF DEATH	CAUSE OF DEATH
Mother	82	Alzheimer's
Father	72	stroke
Sister	76	liver cancer

Murry is a simple man who loves to read
and has worked hard his whole life.

A CELEBRATION OF THEIR
HOMETOWN CENTENARIANS

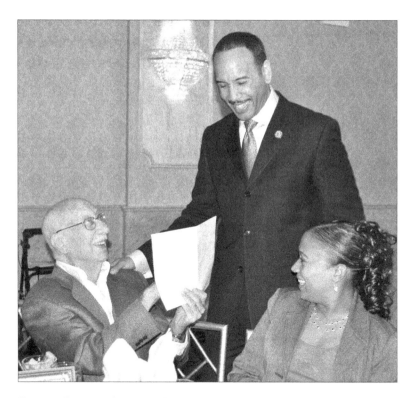

Bronx Borough President Rueben Diaz, Jr. shares a laugh with one of the honorees and subjects in this book, Oscar Chaikin, and guest.

A BRONX TALE

I n an annual tradition, the office of the Bronx Borough President, the Bronx Tourism Council and the Bronx Economic Development Corporation produce a series of exciting Bronx-wide events over an 11-day period celebrating the very best the borough has to offer. "Bronx Week" includes a 7-day film festival, trolley tours, health fairs, environmental programs, the highly-anticipated Bronx Ball and numerous other events hosted by the community, local businesses and the Borough President's office.

Commemorating their beloved centenarians

Bronx Week also honors the borough's cherished centenarians. Each year, the Bronx Borough President commemorates the lives of those "Bronxites" who have turned, or are soon to be turning, 100 years old. A 4-hour-long lavish banquet is held and attended by local centenarians, their guests and local press by invitation only.

In the midst of my search for extraordinary centenarians to feature in *Extraordinary Centenarians in America*, I was fortunate to receive an invitation to this lovely affair. I got to meet and photograph the honorees and arranged to interview a handful of remarkable folks at a later date.

I met the young and charming Borough President, Rueben Diaz, Jr., along with 42 magnetic centenarians. I thought I would find possibly one or two who really stood out from the crowd; those who exuded positive energy and were active and lively. My intention was to interview these select few individuals for the book at a later date to find out their secrets to vibrant longevity.

However, as it turned out, my experience was quite the contrary to my expectations. In fact, it was extremely difficult to choose just

> *Many were
> cutting the rug
> for most of the afternoon
> with no canes, no wheel
> chairs, just with their
> pure joy and
> strong spirit.*

a few because so many of them fit the bill of "extraordinary". Many were cutting the rug for most of the afternoon with no canes, no wheel chairs, just with their pure joy and strong spirit.

I could not believe how many incredibly vital centenarians resided right here in the Bronx. What was it about their lives and lifestyles here that enabled them to do so? Perhaps a contributing factor to their longevity is the multitude of programs and facilities that are available for the elderly in the Bronx. Their comprehensive Senior Citizen Resource Guide includes over 160 senior centers and several other programs developed to enhance the quality of life for seniors. [Other cities could take note of these programs.] Perhaps it was the vast amount of respect and adoration these seniors receive from their local political leaders and community.

Amidst my marathon of mingling while dining, dancing and photographing the event, I found the following individuals, including a few who were unable to attend the event but were strongly recommended by one or more of the honorees. All of these individuals generously shared their lives, lifestyles and lessons to inspire our readers in the pages of *Extraordinary Centenarians in America.*

Barbara Brody	*age*	102
Oscar Chaikin		99
Miriam Henson		105
Loretta Hodge		102
Irving Ladimer		96
Winifred Thomas		101
Sandra Horowitz		97
Hilda Schwall Berner		97
Johanna Zurndorfer		97

As I was exiting the banquet, I was walking beside the family of one of the honorees. They were chatting away about the event and laughing heartily as one daughter yelled out, "Wow, how lucky we are!" That said it all!

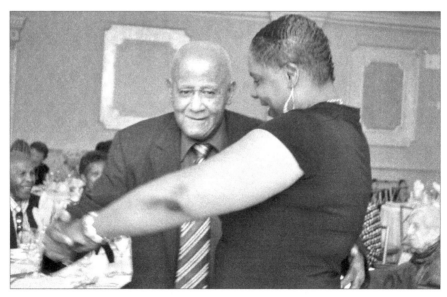

Larcenia Walton, event organizer, with centenarian Alfred C. Moore.

Attorney, Professor, Civic Leader

Born: February 16, 1916, in Manhattan, New York

Current residence: Riverdale, New York

IRVING LADIMER

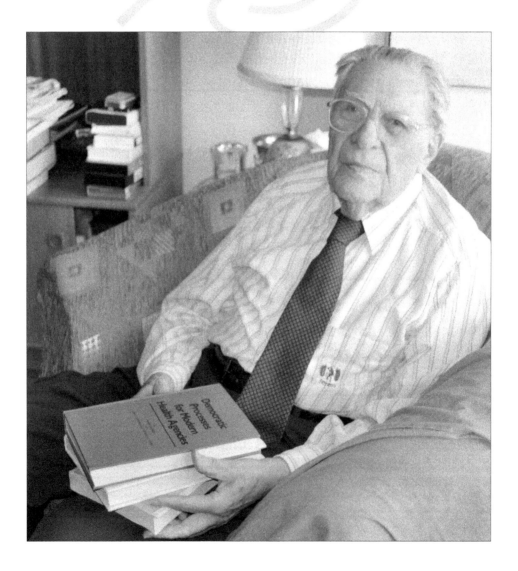

Words of Wisdom

96

"For a long, healthy life, you need a plan and a purpose. It could be family, writing a book, becoming president. Without a purpose, plan or objective, what do you need?"

Mr. Irving Ladimer has been often called the "Mayor of Riverdale" and after meeting this man, I see why. We first met at Schervier, a local Health Services Center in the affluent Riverdale neighborhood within the Bronx in New York City. Irving, formerly a rehab patient at Schervier due to a serious fall, is now their "professional volunteer." Nearly every person who walked by us greeted him with great enthusiasm reflecting his well-deserved popularity. Perhaps this was due to his passionate, unconditional service or maybe his infectious personality.

Irving, a few years short of 100, is one of the most well-rounded, intelligent, witty and supportive individuals I have ever had the pleasure of knowing. Irving's essence is pure goodness. When I contacted this man after hearing about his vibrant life, he not only generously

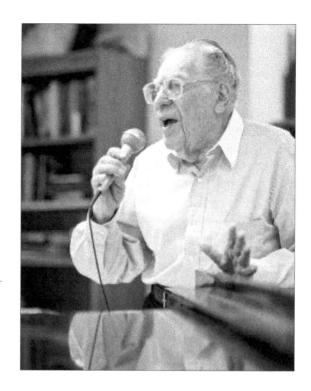

Irving Ladimer, age 96, speaks at Riverdale Senior Services to celebrate the anniversary of the United States constitution. Photo courtesy of Mr Ladimer

agreed to share his story and wisdom with our readers, he wanted to assist me, connect me with other incredible centenarians, and share his vast array of knowledge and experience as an accomplished author. Here are the highlights of this man's incredible life.

A dedicated activist for human rights

Irving is the type of person who always thinks bigger than himself, who always strives to contribute something new and valuable to the world. His high-rise apartment in Riverdale is encumbered with plaques and awards reflecting achievements ranging from Man of the Year, Lifetime Achievement to Leadership in the Jewish Community and more.

An attorney and professor with a specialty in health care issues, Irving has published hundreds of articles on various topics such as patient safety, rights for the elderly, ethics, nutrition, and others. He has written several books and even conducted his own scientific study with his wife on temperament in children. A true thinker, Irving has served as a professor at several colleges (including Yale, Columbia and NYU), conducted studies for the US Public Health Service, American Arbitration Association, Mount Sinai School of

Medicine and the Better Business Bureau (of which he was a vice president at one time).

A week in the life of Irving Ladimer

At 96, Irving is still working as Director of Education and Research for a faculty insurance group, which he founded, helping physicians mostly in medical schools improve doctor-patient relationships and to avoid errors. He typically commutes to Manhattan one day each week producing on-line education regarding medical law and he attends on average four meetings per week for his various associations. He also occasionally speaks to religious groups. On weekends, Irving says, "I see my friends from the community and my girlfriends; you've got to have those!"

Irving spends much of his time volunteering his services for the aging, the legal community and religious community. He is a "professional volunteer" at Schervier, a Catholic Health Services Center, a trustee at his local synagogue and until recently, served as men's club president.

> *"I see my friends from the community and my girlfriends; you've got to have those!"*

Overcoming challenging times

Despite all of his achievements, Irving has had some very challenging times. He lost his first wife, at age 68, after 38 years of marriage and still "misses her dearly." He did remarry and his second wife died after only 11 years. About 15 years ago, Irving's house burned down apparently due to an electrical fire. Fortunately no one was hurt, but Irving was devastated. He is still struggling to adapt to his current space. "It has changed my way of working and thinking. I haven't published in years as the apartment doesn't lend itself to writing."

How does Irving overcome these challenges? Simple, he continues

155

Irving plans to reach out to schools and community centers to teach people of all ages about civics.

to work on making a difference. Irving's current mission is to encourage fellow Americans to become more civic-minded and to get involved in their community. He, and his younger counterpart, 35-year-old State Senator Gustavo Rivera have started campaigns, reaching out to schools and community centers to teach people about the constitution, elections and the government.

I can't wait to see what he's up to next.

REACHING FOR 100 & BEYOND! 96 YEARS

Lifestyle

General health	Irving has never been seriously ill and has had a cold only on rare occasions. He is on no medication and walks with no assistance from a cane or a walker.
Smoking	Never.
Alcohol	Occasional wine.
Nutrition	Irving's wives always cooked whole, natural foods with vegetables and occasionally meats. He was never overweight, but was underweight in his early years. Currently, he eats "some vegetables, fruit, starch, protein and dessert occasionally, has soups and salads, tea or coffee and juice, nothing fancy, nothing excessive." He takes Vitamin D and iron regularly.
Physical activity	Irving had no specific athletic interest but was "always on the go, walking all the time."

Current interests	Irving avidly reads the *The New York Times*, magazines, legal and medical journals, occasionally books, *The New Yorker* short stories; "reading is a very important part of my life—for enjoyment and analysis." When Irving travels, he typically visits the library to research if there is anyone he knows living in the area. Irving also maintains a large circle of academic friends from NY, Chicago, Washington, DC, and Boston, from the synagogue and his volunteer work.
Family	Irving is very close with his 2 daughters, who are in their 60s. They live out of state but he speaks with them regularly. He sees his cousin in Manhattan every few weeks and he also has a house in Singer Island, Florida. He has no siblings.

Family history

	AGE OF DEATH	CAUSE OF DEATH
Mother	88	natural causes
Father	89	accident

Irving is one of the most well-rounded, intelligent, witty and supportive individuals I have ever met.

Survivor, Caregiver, Advocate For The Needy
Born: October 21, 1915, in Germany (immigrated in 1936)
Current residence: Riverdale, New York

JOHANNA ZURNDORFER

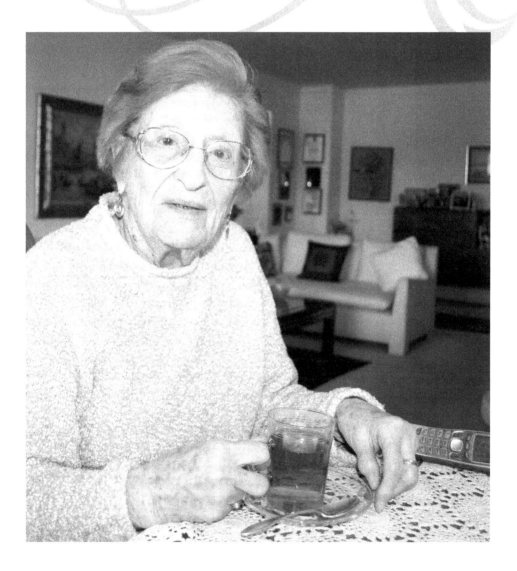

Words of Wisdom

97

*"Do what you
have to do.
Don't analyze it,
just do it."*

Just 20 years old, Johanna Zurndorfer immigrated to America with absolutely no money; she was running for her life.

Johanna came from a lovely bucolic village in the Black Forest of southern Germany called Rexingen. In 1650, the first two Jewish families settled there after fleeing the Chmielnicki massacres in Poland. Subsequently, Jews from other countries settled at this small village and established a strong and thriving Jewish community into the 1930s. Johanna was witness to the beginning of the demise of her precious hometown.

As a young woman, Johanna traveled back and forth to Frankfurt daily where she worked as an apprentice for a bookkeeper. Says Johanna, "You needed to be an apprentice for three years before you could get any work." Although, she described her small village as

> *"We couldn't go to the movies anymore. When we went for a walk on Shabbat, they threw stones at us."*

idyllic and peaceful, she started noticing a movement of anti-Semitism rising in Frankfurt. As it spread, Johanna describes, "We couldn't go to the movies anymore. When we went for a walk on Shabbat, they threw stones at us."

Her family noticed many people starting to emigrate, anticipating that it would get worse as Hitler gained more power and momentum. However, there was a limit on the number of refugees allowed into America. Johanna said, "It was like the lottery, in order to get a visa, you had to have a certain number. If your number was too high, you could not get into America. My family was lucky as we all were able to get out in time. Many people were stuck in Germany and sent to (concentration) camps."

Some of Johanna's neighbors formed a group of about 40 and immigrated to Israel. They were joined by others from nearby towns and, in 1938, founded what is called the Shavei Zion settlement. Just a few months later, the interior of the synagogue back in

> *"We all were able to get out. Many people were stuck in Germany and sent to (concentration) camps."*

Rexingen was destroyed. In 1939, the 126 Jews left in the town were deported and only three survived. All that remains of the once flourishing community is the cemetery, the synagogue building that has been converted into a church, and a memorial that was built for the concentration camp victims. A damaged Torah scroll from Rexingen is preserved in a memorial hall in Shavei Zion.

The village of Rexingen has become somewhat famous since a book was published recently by one of the villagers' children. Johanna pulled this book from her coffee table and placed it in my hands. She said, "Do you see that little girl on the cover? That is me."

160

Life in America

Indeed, Johanna and her family escaped almost certain death; however, life was not easy when they arrived in America, landing right in the midst of the Great Depression. Although unemployment was at its peak and Johanna was brand new to this country, she still managed to land a job as a maid on Amsterdam Avenue in Manhattan. She'd survived the worst nightmare of her life with her family intact; it seemed that the rest of life's obstacles would be a breeze.

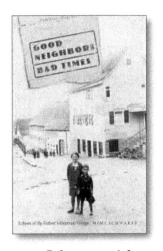

Johanna with a neighbor on the cover of a book describing the plight of her beloved hometown village, Rexingen

Fate has it, after living in Manhattan for four years, Johanna met the man she would be married to for the next 54 years. And, as they say, "birds of a feather…" the love of her life unbelievably came from her beloved village of Rexingen! Shortly thereafter, her husband went into the Army and she went to work at a pocketbook factory.

As more obstacles came her way, Johanna just took them on like a veteran survivor. After he graduated college, her only son was diagnosed with Multiple Sclerosis. She took care of him for years while she worked as a bookkeeper part-time, until he eventually passed away at only 52. Her only daughter was also diagnosed with MS years later and at 65 is still struggling with it. Married for 30 years, Johanna's husband then suffered from a terrible stroke. He was functional, but had trouble speaking. Johanna was his caregiver as well for 20 years until his death 16 years ago. When asked how she dealt with all of this hardship, Johanna says humbly, "Life was not easy, but it made me stronger."

> "Life was not easy, but it made me stronger."

Still giving in her senior years

After years of working and caring for her family through many rough times, Johanna is still actively giving and making a difference for others. In her late 90s, Johanna still visits the MS center every week, as she has been doing for over 25 years, and has formed a group at her synagogue that reaches out to people in need on a daily basis. She is very active in the community, has been called a "community leader and organizer" by others and maintains many close friendships. Johanna loves to play bridge, does her own laundry and taxes, goes to Bible class regularly and the beauty parlor, and still drives to visit friends and family. Her health is still good, although she has lost sight in one eye.

That small village benevolence instilled in her since she was a child, Johanna makes sure to visit her Jewish community each Friday evening to wish them a good "Shabbos" [a day of rest and worship in the Jewish religion].

REACHING FOR 100 & BEYOND! 97 YEARS

Lifestyle

Smoking	Occasional cigarette.
Alcohol	Occasional drink.
Nutrition	"A healthy diet of balanced home-cooked meals most of my life" although Johanna was approximately 30 lbs. overweight until she was in her 50s. Subsequently, she moderated her intake and has never been overweight since. She never took vitamins.

Physical activity	Never formally exercised, but was always active and "on the go."
Current interests	Weekly visits to the Multiple Sclerosis Center for 25 years to volunteer. Formed a group that calls less fortunate people for support every afternoon from her temple. Plays bridge, goes to Bible class, visits other Jewish people to wish them "Shabbat shalom" and meets friends for lunch. Still does her laundry and taxes and goes to the beauty parlor weekly.
Family	Sees family regularly and enjoys lots of friends. She has her one surviving daughter, one granddaughter and two great-grandchildren. Although she's lost all of her old friends, she's met many new ones through her temple.

Family history

	AGE OF DEATH	CAUSE OF DEATH
Mother	101	natural causes
Father	62	heart failure, heavy smoker
Half-Sister*	72	cancer
Half-Sister*	68	cancer
Half-Brother*	35	complications from surgery/epileptic
Son	52	Multiple Sclerosis**

*Father's side

**Daughter has MS and was diagnosed in her 40s. She is now 65 years old.

Nanny, Housekeeper (For Bette Davis And Patrick O'Neal)
Born: June 26, 1910, in St. Thomas, Virgin Islands
Current residence: Bronx, NY

LORETTA HODGE

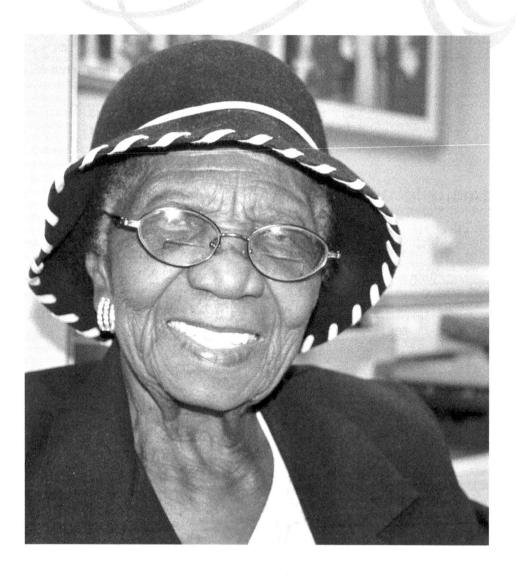

Words of Wisdom

102

"Whatever is hard, you make hard, but if you take it as it comes, it doesn't come hard. Don't worry, don't want so much, and be satisfied with what you've got. Be willing to share with your friends and those less fortunate."

Chatting briefly with Ms. Loretta Hodge, a 102-year old honoree I met at the Bronx Centenarian Gala, I asked what her advice would be for younger individuals to lead a long, vibrant life. She immediately quipped, donning a huge, playful grin, "Have lots of sex!"

Living life to the fullest

Loretta had the liveliest eyes and when she spoke, her smile lit up her face and mine. This was a lady I wished to know better.

A few weeks later, I visited Loretta at a rehab facility in the Bronx which she was attending temporarily as she had recently broken her hip. However, sitting around for rehab was too much of a bore for Loretta. Soon after she arrived, she began partaking in a myriad

> "We took a journey on a boat for 5 days to get to the United States. It wasn't too rough though, we partied every day."

of activities available at the resident daycare center. This center was for seniors who are living at home, but who could still benefit from a life-enhancing, structured day and supportive community environment, and this is exactly what Loretta desired.

Facing challenges with grace and gratitude

Loretta was born in St. Thomas, Virgin Islands. Her parents, whom she barely knew, left her to be raised by her beloved godmother, who died when Loretta was just 15 years old. Before her godmother died, she taught Loretta many lessons, including one she would never forget and would incorporate into her life forever: "Always take life as it comes and it will never seem hard."

Since childhood, Loretta's dream was to live in America as she heard from her friends that it was a wonderful place where "everyone was dressed up all the time." So, after saving up enough of her earnings from various jobs in domestic work, Loretta left her hometown to pursue her dream. She moved to Harlem, New York to live with her sister. She was 24 years old, completely alone on her journey, and never looked back. Loretta recalls, "We took a journey on a boat for 5 days to get to

> "They were paying 25 cents an hour. I grabbed a job where the woman said I would make $1.50 for cleaning just two windows. She even took me out for a cup of coffee. However, when I asked why she just paid me only $1.25, she told me that she took out 25 cents for the coffee!"

the United States. It wasn't too rough though, we partied every day."

Unfortunately, it wasn't the best of times in America when Loretta arrived as it was during the heart of the Great Depression. Loretta was flustered. The only people she saw dressed up were those gentleman selling pencils and apples on the street. "It was strange in the beginning as there were these men hollering outside every day selling fish and vegetables. It was not at all what I expected!"

Loretta married and lived in an apartment for $1.50 a month. She bore five children, although three of them died in infancy, as they were premature. Her husband eventually went off to serve in the military during WWII and was killed while on duty. And, her beloved sister, at only 35 years old, passed away from complications from the flu.

> "Domestic work wasn't so easy then, as it is now. They didn't have any vacuum cleaners. You would have to pull up the rugs and hit them with a broom to get the dust out. You didn't have a mop, just a rubber towel and would have to wipe the floors by hand with a pail of water."

Loretta was left alone again, but this time with her two boys. She needed to work, so she hired someone to watch her children while she took care of others. At the same time, she participated in the church choir (one of her fondest memories) where she happily sang for 53 years surrounded by friends and neighbors. Many of those choir members and spectators still call and visit her these days in her Bronx apartment.

Domestic bliss?

Loretta would wait on the street hoping to get picked for a job in housekeeping. "They were paying 25 cents an hour. I grabbed a job where the woman said I would make $1.50 for cleaning just two windows. She even took me out for a cup of coffee. However, when I asked why she just paid me only $1.25, she told me that she took out $.25 for the coffee!"

Loretta took various jobs living in and out as a nanny and housekeeper, making $40 a month in the post-war era. "At one live-in job I never had to buy underwear or stockings because the little child I was watching told his parents that he wouldn't eat unless they would buy me what I needed."

"Domestic work wasn't so easy then, as it is now. They didn't have any vacuum cleaners. You would have to pull up the rugs and hit them with a broom to get the dust out. You didn't have a mop, just a rubber towel and would have to wipe the floors by hand with a pail of water." However, Loretta was grateful for what she had, as not having to pay for rent or food was a big plus during this time.

> "Bette Davis was so different from what you would expect from a well-known celebrity. She often offered me tea and gave me money to buy presents for myself and my children for Easter."

Changing Bette Davis's bed sheets

By far, the most extraordinary job experience for Loretta was working for actor Patrick O'Neal and his wife Cynthia. Loretta's memory is so impeccable, she even recalled O'Neal's address at the time, over 50 years ago, on 108th and Lexington Avenue. She took care of their two adopted sons and cleaned the house. During that time, O'Neal was appearing on Broadway in the popular play, *Night of the Iguana*, with Bette Davis. Ms. Davis came to live with them while performing in the show. Loretta said, "Bette Davis was so different from what you would expect from a famous celebrity. She often offered me tea and gave me money to buy presents for myself and my children for Easter."

A survivor, a giver

Loretta worked in domestic care most of her life. After retiring, she continued going to church every Sunday and for special events. She would also regularly visit sick people and give some of her things to the less fortunate. "I want to share, it makes you strong. Not wanting a whole lot makes you feel satisfied. When you are not envious, you are more satisfied."

She is hoping to walk again soon after physical therapy so she can get back to helping others again. Although she could walk with the assistance of a "walker" following her injury, that's not acceptable to her and she is striving to walk independently once again.

Loretta had never been in a hospital until just last year when she broke her hip. Her memory is sharp, her skin should belong to a woman 30 years younger, and her spirit seems even younger. Just her presence would brighten your day.

> "I want to share, it makes you strong. Not wanting a whole lot makes you feel satisfied. When you are not envious, you are more satisfied."

> "Many of the people I have met and helped over the years, now call, visit me and help me out occasionally, and that is a great comfort to me."

Loretta attributes her longevity to a "happy-go-lucky attitude and an ability to get accustomed to life's challenges. You get along with people by being kind and helpful."

Loretta has four grandchildren and ten great-grandchildren. Presently, she lives in her own apartment in the Bronx with help from one of her sons (who are presently 73 and 75). She admittedly loves men. She often jokes around and tells strangers that her son is her boyfriend and that she enjoys having a male aide.

In closing, Loretta quips, "I had a good life. I don't like old men and I like plenty of sex! Once I lose one man, I look for a younger man…. Just joking."

REACHING 100 & BEYOND! 102 YEARS

Lifestyle

General health	Loretta was always healthy with no serious illnesses.
Smoking	Up until her 20s but could not afford it anymore, so she quit.
Alcohol	Occasionally on a weekend or at a special occasion.
Nutrition	"I never ate much—now it's tea and toast for breakfast, salmon with rice for lunch, chicken for dinner." In her earlier years, Loretta cooked all of her meals, all natural whole foods, vegetables (broccoli, spinach, carrots), some chicken, pork chops and meatloaf. She was never overweight. "When you are so busy, you don't have time to eat a lot."
Physical activity	No regimen but was always active due to the nature of her job.
Current interests	Going to church every week, a variety of activities at the senior center.
Family	Loretta has 4 grandchildren and 10 great-grandchildren, although she hardly sees them. She sees one of her two sons regularly, but she still lives independently.

Family history

	AGE OF DEATH	CAUSE OF DEATH
Mother	unknown	unknown
Father	unknown	unknown
Sister	35	complications from the flu

She immediately quipped,
donning a huge, playful grin,
"Have lots of sex!"

Salesman, Business Owner, Caulbearer

Born: December 24, 1912, in Bronx, New York

Current residence: Yonkers, New York

OSCAR CHAIKIN

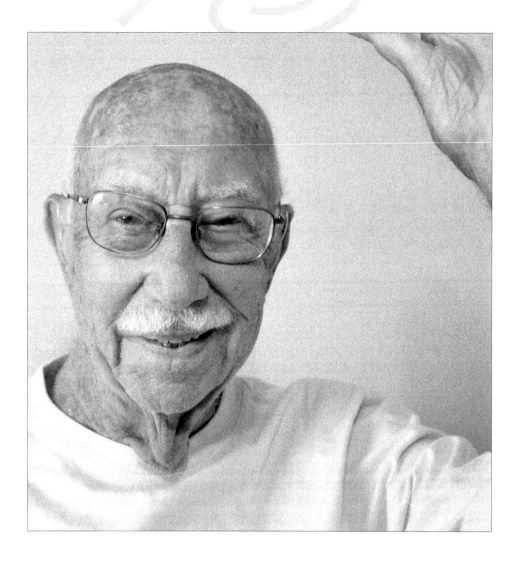

Words of Wisdom

99

"I've always been thin and active, but I also have been really lucky, as I was born in a sac!"

I sat across from Mr. Oscar Chaikin at the Bronx Centenarian Tribute. He is a sturdy man with a big smile, not fragile in the least, particularly for a man of 99. As it was quite loud at this lively event, Oscar agreed to meet with me at a later date to share his words of wisdom at his charming home at the Classic Residence, a beautiful continuing care retirement center (CCRC).

Protected by a "sac"?

Oscar Chaikin was quite the anomaly. While he does have a few things in common with the other vibrant seniors profiled in this book, he truly pushed the envelope when it came to his health and well-being.

For one, Oscar smoked cigarettes regularly until he was 85,

> ## "My mother always told me, 'you will always be lucky as you were born in a sac'."

drank a glass of Scotch daily for decades and grew up eating so much of his grandmother's fried food, he eventually developed an ulcer. So how did he get so old?

First, it must be noted that after developing the ulcer in his 20s, Oscar was much more careful about what he consumed, avoiding fried food and bread, and never allowed himself to become overweight. He was also very active physically and always remained mentally active. However, Oscar had his own theory regarding his extreme longevity.

Says Oscar, "I always go back to what my mother told me when I was a little boy. She said, 'You will always be lucky as you were born in a sac.' The sac Oscar refers to is also known as a caul (pronounced cowl), or birth veil. It is, in reality, the amniotic sac, but in this case the baby was born with the sac still around it. Those born with a caul are called caulbearers. In medieval times, the appearance of a caul on a newborn was seen as a sign of good luck.

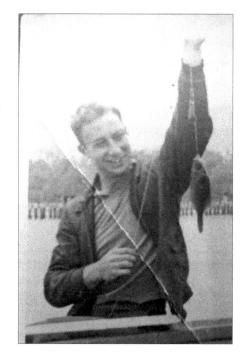

Oscar says he is lucky at fishing and in life generally, but can't make predictions like the caulbearers of ancient times. Photo courtesy of Oscar Chaikin

174

Such births are extremely rare. It has been calculated that caulbearer births may be as few as one in eighty thousand births and they hold special significance for the child born in such a manner. Additionally, most caulbearers are born with the sac around their faces only (hence the term 'birth veil'), whereas in Oscar's case, it encased his entire body like a cocoon.

Traditions say that caulbearers can predict when weather patterns will change, are true leaders, and have extraordinary insight amongst other abilities. In the day, many could predict when fish and other food supplies would become plentiful. According to Oscar, he did love to fish, but did not possess any of these abilities. However, he was indeed lucky.

Besides being generally healthy during his long life despite all of the smoking and drinking, Oscar provided me with an example of how his luck started at such an early age, which he attributed to this mysterious phenomenon. "I was 3 years old and rode my tricycle down a full flight of stairs. For one, I was lucky to survive that, but later on my mother discovered a huge black mark on my leg. They thought it was a clot, rushed me to the hospital where they discovered it was gangrene. In those days, they would certainly have to amputate my leg given the amount of gangrene, but they somehow found a way to remove all of it and save my leg." Due to this injury, which hindered him just a bit physically, he was able to avoid being drafted into the Army during WWII.

> "I got a part-time job at night making 75 cents an hour and they gave me 35 cents for dinner. When I didn't have work, I would still get dressed and pretend to go so that my mother would accept the money I had saved up."

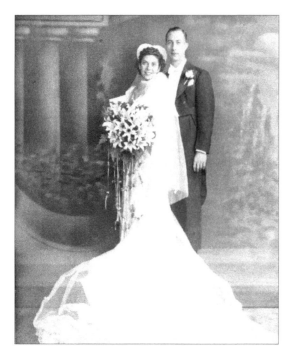

Rose and Oscar's wedding day.
Photo courtesy of Nancy Chaikin

A remarkable man during difficult times

As a young man, Oscar was always very responsible, saving up his money for a "rainy day." It was a good thing as there were many of those "rainy days" soon to come. During the Great Depression, his money came in handy for the family. Although working regularly prior to it, once the Great Depression hit its full stride, Oscar could not get a full-time job.

"I got a part-time job at night making 75 cents an hour and they gave me 35 cents for dinner. When I didn't have work, I would still get dressed and pretend to go so that my mother would accept the money I had saved up."

Fortunately, his dad got them through the Depression and became quite successful, as he was the only man in New York City who could repair the radiators for the Model T Fords.

Standing on his injury his entire life

Although he had a leg injury, Oscar never had a job working at a desk. He worked on his feet his entire life. He initially worked as a salesman and subsequently owned a successful hardware store in Manhattan for over 40 years. There, he was also on his feet the entire day. "I didn't let the leg bother me. My legs are very strong today because of how often I used them." He worked six days a week and retired at 62 years old.

What a great pair!

Oscar met his beloved wife, Rose, when he was a teenager. She lived right down the street in his Bronx neighborhood. Says Nancy, Oscar's daughter, "My parents were a great pair. In their youth, she was as beautiful as he was handsome. As a married couple, they both loved nothing more than being with family and friends—of which they had many. All of them lived in the same neighborhood."

"I was always fit. I used to dance more, and I used to have a lot of muscles. Now I am lucky that I have skin!"

Nancy adds, "My parents were the life of many a party. Once they were offered a summer bungalow for free because everyone had such fun when they were around. They were great dancers of the cha-cha and mambo and once won a dance contest as 'Oscar and Yolanda'."

"My dad was a storyteller and knew a good joke for any occasion, liked a fine Scotch and a cigar, laughed heartily at his own and others' good jokes and respected people for their good deeds and values. My mom, Rosie, was the perfect hostess—she threw theme parties including luaus—long before Martha Stewart and party stores existed."

On Rose's 85th birthday, Oscar gave her original sheet music for *My Dear Old Rose*. On it, he inscribed, "I was lucky to get the only 'Rose' that never faded."

Oscar was happily married to Rose for 65 years. She died 8 years ago at 88.

Staying active in his elder years

Since Rose's passing, Oscar has lived alone and independently, aside from his two beloved parakeets and assistance from an aide, in a bustling retirement community where he remains very active. He goes to Yonkers Raceway monthly, plays cards weekly and participates at every family function, dancing through the night. He keeps his mind active by reading the newspaper daily and listening to classical music.

Every year for the last 20+ years, Oscar has spent the entire summer in New Hampshire with his son's family, enjoying his son, his grandchildren and the ocean. He has his own guesthouse; a renovated calf barn the family calls 'the nest', short for the 'love nest' back when his wife was alive.

REACHING FOR 100 & BEYOND! *99* YEARS

Lifestyle

General health	Besides an ulcer, Oscar has remained healthy his entire life.
Smoking	Until he was 85.
Alcohol	A shot of Dewar's Scotch every day—Oscar believed that alcohol killed germs. "The doctors never had meds then like they have now, but those meds contained lots of alcohol!"
Nutrition	In the early part of his life, his grandmother cooked and it was often fried and laden with fat. After developing an ulcer around age 27, Oscar became more conscious of what he ate, avoiding fried foods and reducing his consumption of bread. He consumed very little vegetables and ate various meats, but very moderate portions. He has remained trim his entire life.

Physical activity	Oscar has always been active, working 6 days a week on his feet helping customers and always stayed fit, although he did not have a structured fitness regimen. He also loves to dance.
Currrent interests	Oscar loves reading, listening to classical music, going to the racetrack, playing cards at his community, dancing through the night and spending lots of time with his family.
Family	One daughter and two sons, 7 granddaughters and 9 great-grandchildren who visit him regularly. Looks forward to spending every summer at his eldest son's house in New Hampshire with his two parakeets. Lives with the help of an aide.

Family history

	AGE OF DEATH	CAUSE OF DEATH
Mother	59	high blood pressure
Father	70	n/a
Brother	n/a	living, age 96
Brother	97	heart attack
Brother	85	complication from surgery
Brother	61	complication from prescription drugs

Oscar happily smoked cigarettes, drank Scotch daily and ate fried food.

Secretary, Community Leader

Born: March 29, 1915, in Boston, Massachusetts

Current residence: Bronx, New York

HILDA SCHWALL BERNER

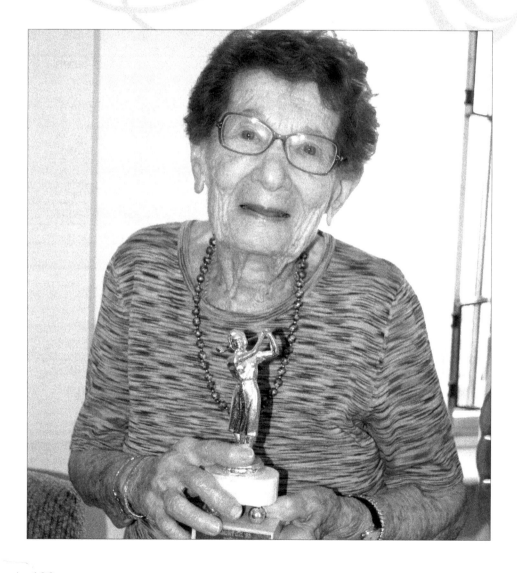

Words of Wisdom

97

"Try to understand the kind of person you are and accept who you are; but if you want to improve your situation, change it. Keep your eye on the stars and try to succeed at what you want to do."

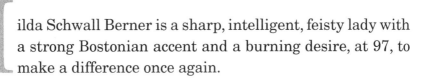

ilda Schwall Berner is a sharp, intelligent, feisty lady with a strong Bostonian accent and a burning desire, at 97, to make a difference once again.

A Bostonian through and through

Hilda was born and bred in Boston and proud of it. "I grew up there, went to college there, got married and raised my children there." She met her husband, Bob, while she was in high school and he was in college. They married when Hilda was 24, and had two children, a son and a daughter. They were married for 56 years until Bob died at age 91. Hilda described him as "the most wonderful husband and father you would ever want to know."

"As a teenager, I remember trying to scrape up money just to go to the movies, but my friends and I were all in the same boat. I also remember my parents discussing whether or not they could afford to buy me a winter coat."

Managing hard times

The Great Depression took its toll on Hilda and her family, but they still managed better than most. "As a teenager, I remember trying to scrape up money just to go to the movies, but my friends and I were all in the same boat. I also remember my parents discussing whether or not they could afford to buy me a winter coat. My father was actually a furrier and I ended up getting a coat made from a member of the skunk family. One snowy day, I was wearing it to school and hung it up in the coatroom. The entire room smelled of my coat. I was very embarrassed to say the least. I had to wait a long time for the mink."

Hilda was accepted to the all-girls school called Simmons College, which is now co-ed. She actually had to take a 'tennis test' as part of the application process for the college. After graduating, Hilda was quite busy. She took a job as a secretary in a furniture manufacturing business, subsequently worked for a direct mail advertising association, once again worked as a secretary at Lansberg's Department Store and finally worked for her husband in mergers and acquisitions until she retired at 60.

"I feel the world is much more dangerous now. There is too much violence and too many guns out there."

182

Politics and community leadership

Although Hilda left her various paid vocations, she retired to a busy life of community service and politics. She was an honorary life trustee of United Jewish Appeal (UJA), and member of the League of Women Voters, Beth Israel Hospital and various other organizations. Earlier, Hilda was elected to the Brookline Town Meeting, proudly serving alongside Michael Dukakis well before he became Governor of Massachusetts and later the Democratic candidate for President of the United States.

Hilda moved to Florida and lived independently. She played golf avidly until she was 94. "I have several trophies to prove it!" She surrounded herself with many close friends in a wonderful community.

Just a few years ago, Hilda moved to a beautiful senior retirement facility in the Bronx. There she participates in various structured activities; however, she feels adamant that she can be making more of a difference. Says Hilda, "I feel the world is much more dangerous now. There is too much violence and too many guns out there."

Hilda's advice to the younger generation: "Be and do the best that you can. If you are unhappy about something, take action and try to improve it." She still follows this mantra and will no doubt keep on trying to make a difference no matter what situation and no matter what age.

Hilda's mother, father and sister all passed away at the age of 76. When she visited her physician as she approached that dreadful

> *"Be and do the best that you can. If you are unhappy about something, take action and try to improve it."*

183

number, she asked him if she would be meeting the same fate. The physician advised her, "Don't worry, the way you are going, you will reach 100." At 97, it seems that is one more goal she intends on reaching.

REACHING FOR 100 & BEYOND! 97 YEARS

Lifestyle

General health	Excellent her entire life, just recently on medication for her heart.
Smoking	Hilda tried smoking in college but did not enjoy it. She never smoked again.
Alcohol	An occasional drink.
Nutrition	Hilda loved healthy home-cooked, mostly "low key American meals"; chicken soup, chicken, some challah, gefilte fish, always fresh vegetables, moderate portions of kosher meat. She was of medium build and has been about 7 or 8 pounds overweight at times.
Physical activity	In her earlier years, Hilda played tennis. After she married, she became a serious golfer until she was 94, winning several trophies at interclub matches. Until recently, she was walking every day for 30 to 45 minutes.
Current interests	Follows politics and is an avid reader. Participates in some activities at her retirement community but much less in recent years.

Family	Hilda's son calls her every day and sees her every weekend. She also sees her daughter on a more infrequent basis. She has 5 grandchildren.

Family history

	AGE OF DEATH	CAUSE OF DEATH
Mother	76	heart attack
Father	76	heart attack
Sibling	76	n/a
Sibling	n/a	living, age 85

Hilda is a sharp, intelligent, feisty lady with a strong Bostonian accent and a burning desire to make a difference.

Homemaker, Caretaker, Retail Clerk
Born: March 20, 1907, in Georgia
Current residence: Bronx, New York

MIRIAM HENSON

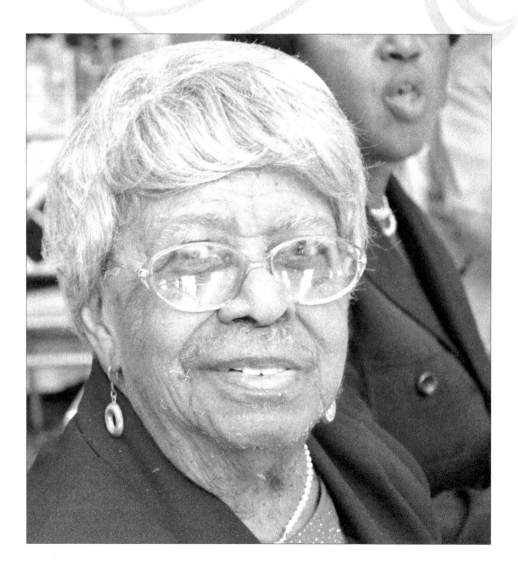

Words of Wisdom

105

"You must keep active or you will just wither away. Always be involved in some activity."

I had the pleasure of meeting Ms. Miriam Henson at the Bronx Centenarian Tribute Gala. I noticed this energetic woman on the dance floor. She was impeccably dressed, perfectly coiffed, and 'cutting the rug' with some of the other guests. I wondered if she could actually be one of the honored centenarians? Indeed, this charming, soft-spoken woman was 104 years old at the time. She wasn't even out of breath! Being active is her credo and it has served her well.

I chatted with Ms. Henson briefly and she agreed to reveal her secrets for her vibrant longevity at a separate time, in a quieter environment, at her home in Co-op City.

Growing up after the Great War

Born in the State of Georgia, Miriam and her family moved to New

York when she was a child in 1918, just after World War I had come to an end. Young Miriam was excited about the end of the war. She recalled Armistice Day when "there were parades everywhere!" When asked about her experience living through WWI, Miriam says, "I was so young that I didn't understand it much, but when I went to the store to buy a loaf of bread for a nickel and the store clerk asked for a penny more, it was my first experience of how the war affected the economy."

"When I went to the store to buy a loaf of bread for a nickel and the store clerk asked for a penny more, it was my first experience of how the war affected the economy."

"When the Great Depression began, it was quite the opposite. There was never enough food. I would go to the store and often there was nothing left because some people would just buy all of it. You would have to get up at 5 a.m. before they took everything. One day all the meat and chicken were gone and all there was left was duck—I didn't know how to cook duck!"

Miriam spoke extensively about the difference between the mentalities of people back then versus now. "People nowadays say how [the state of the economy] is the worst thing that ever happened to them but they are just not used to what we had to live through. We are used to so much war and poverty. I think unemployment [insurance benefits] hurts people from getting new jobs as they feel they can stay on it until they get

"Nowadays some people just stay on unemployment and don't try as hard to get another job."

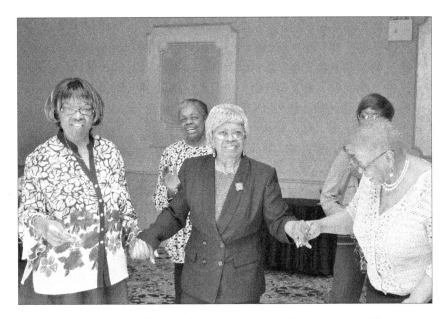

Miriam Henson, 105, celebrating with
some of the younger folk.

back to what they had before. We didn't have that, so it made us take any job that we could get. Nowadays some people just stay on unemployment and don't try as hard to get another job. Additionally, in those days, you had to go to class and learn to be polite and courteous, unlike today."

Managing great loss

Miriam was very close to her mother. When her mother became ill from cancer, Miriam and her husband took her into their home and cared for her for 10 years until she passed. After she died, Miriam was overcome with grief, but instead of allowing the grief to consume her, she managed to get a job, in her 50s, in retail. She worked at Macy's and subsequently Bloomingdale's. This kept her busy, distracted from her grief and around other people.

Years later, Miriam's husband wanted to move to Co-op City, one of the largest cooperative housing developments in the world, situated along the Hutchinson River in the Bronx. This complex was termed "a city within a city" as they had their own schools, supermarkets, doctors and other services, making it virtually unnecessary to leave. However, there was a maximum income allowance to be eligible to live there and Miriam made the couple ineligible as she was making too much money working at Bloomingdale's. A devoted and loving wife, Miriam decided to retire so that her husband could have his wish to live in Co-op City. They were very happy living there and happily married for 43 years until her husband passed away as well.

I formed a group called the 'Retirees' – we would exercise, go on the bus to the beach, walk around Co-op City, play cards and board games."

Fortunately for Miriam, Co-op City had a very large elderly population and its Senior Services Program had many services for its aging citizens. It was actually considered the largest Naturally Occurring Retirement Community (NORC) in the nation.

Miriam, not one to sit around and feel sorry for herself, took full advantage of this. She utilized, and still does, an inexpensive transportation service to get around for practical and social purposes.

If it doesn't exist, create it!

Miriam was always an initiator, a trait that has served her well for close to a century. When she first moved to New York, there were no

Protestant churches for her to pray. So, she gathered a few other Protestants and founded one. When she lived in Queens, there was no bridge club; hence, she started one.

In her later years, after retiring, Miriam explains, "I formed a group called the 'Retirees'—we would exercise, go on the bus to the beach, walk around Co-op City, play cards and board games." Once a month the Retirees would have a social and Miriam would charge money to subsidize the next one.

In her 80s, Miriam was travelling around the world with her friends from the church, through a local organization and with her family. Her last trip was on the *Queen Mary* with her niece when she was 101. "We just missed the earthquake in Turkey that year."

Every decade in her later years, Miriam's large family would throw her a big party. Jokingly, she says, "when I reached 100, I told them, 'you all did your part, now it's my turn'." She chose the destination and spearheaded the celebration herself.

Miriam still lives completely independently, pays her own bills "on time", manages her own checking account, prepares her own food and keeps her own house. She has no aid except some occasional assistance from one of her relatives.

> In her 80s, she was travelling around the world with her friends from the church. Her last trip was on the *Queen Mary* with her niece when she was 101. "We just missed the earthquake in Turkey that year."

Lifestyle

General health	Miriam's health was always excellent except for a minor thyroid operation and hysterectomy. At 105, she has an impeccable memory and perfect hearing.
Smoking	Not since she was a teen as she didn't care for it.
Alcohol	Occasionally port wine with lunch or dinner and occasionally a rum cola.
Nutrition	Miriam was a "small eater" and never heavy. "I was the thin one; my sister and daughter were the chubby ones." She likes rice and vegetables, sometimes salads, does not snack and eats 3 meals a day. "When I'm not hungry, I don't eat any more."
Physical activity	"I was always a Tomboy, loved baseball and I still do. I was always active running after my daughter." Miriam still walks the beach around her neighborhood regularly and was active when she would travel.
Current interests	In her 80s, Miriam traveled the world.
Family	Miriam had one daughter, Virginia, who passed away about 20 years ago, and has many nieces, grandnieces and nephews in other boroughs. On special occasions the whole family gathers together.

Family history

	AGE OF DEATH	CAUSE OF DEATH
Mother	60s	cancer
Father	58	stomach disorder
Brother	70s	unknown
Sister	80s	unknown
Daughter	67	colon cancer

When I noticed this energetic woman on the dance floor, she was 'cutting the rug' with some of the other guests and not even out of breath!

Singer, Actress, Artist, Teacher

Born: June 5, 1909, in Brooklyn, New York

Current residence: Bronx, New York

BARBARA BRODY

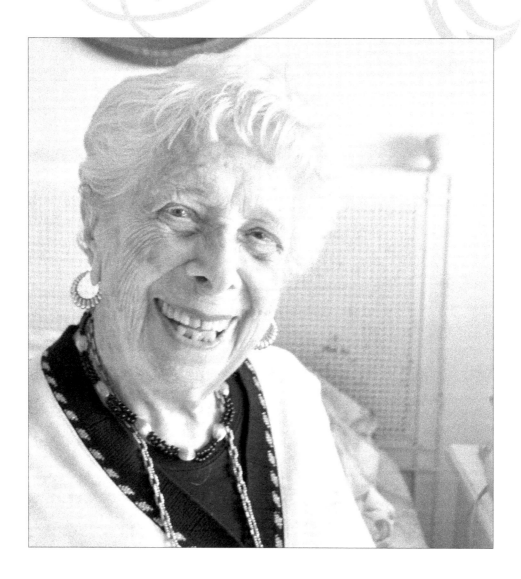

Words of Wisdom

102

*"You have to make
the best out of your life
and have a good attitude."*

The first thing I noticed in Barbara Brody's charming apartment was the wide assortment of lovely, unique paintings and pen and ink drawings. All of them, I soon discovered, were created from Ms. Brody's deft hands and mind's eye.

A woman of the arts

Barbara started painting back in college at New York University, and it became her ongoing passion for most of her life. A woman of the arts, Barbara also loved to sing and act, and was extremely proficient at these as well. After graduating from high school, she studied acting under some very prestigious teachers; however, her parents, being ultra-conservative, did not think it appropriate for Barbara to perform onstage. They didn't like the idea of her going to college either, not uncommon thinking for parents of young girls in those days. Fortunately for Barbara, her more liberal-minded uncle persuaded them to let her go.

Some years later, Barbara was offered a coveted opportunity to train in London for singing and acting, but again, her parents would not permit her to go.

Adamantly refusing to let her parents quell her passion and ambition, Barbara managed her way to star in a Gilbert and Sullivan play as soon as she was finally on her own. She also auditioned for various choruses and sang under the acclaimed Italian conductor Arturo Toscanini at the Metropolitan Opera.

"When Mom was in her 30s and 40s, she would create invitations from rice paper before anyone thought of it, and she sold them. She was interested in everything, all the time. She still sang while she was raising us, but in the temple choir."
– Barbara's daughter, Maris

A devoted daughter and mother

Barbara married her husband, Arthur, when she was 29 and raised two children in her 30s, almost unheard of in those days as most women had children in their late teens or twenties. She decided to end her career in the arts and devote her life to taking care of her children and her ailing parents. Her mother passed away in her 50s of heart disease and her father came to live with them.

However, Barbara was still exercising her creative skills. According to her daughter Maris, who is currently 72, "When mom was in her 30s and 40s, she would create invitations from rice paper before anyone

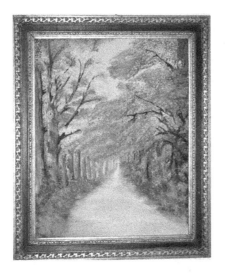

One of Barbara Brody's many original paintings.

thought of it, and she sold them. She was interested in everything, all the time. She still sang while she was raising us, but in the temple choir." Barbara also loved sculpting; some of her pieces still reside with her greatest admirers, her family.

Purpose and wonder in her golden and platinum years

When the children were grown, and she was already in her 50s, Barbara refused to stay idle. She utilized her college degree and went back to work in Manhattan as an elementary school teacher for over 15 years. After she retired, she and Arthur moved to Florida. Maris says, "They were both so curious and educated, they just travelled the world and marveled at it. And, they were both wonderful parents who loved their family."

> "I try not to make a big fuss over things. I always said this too shall pass."

When Barbara was not travelling, she took courses in art and in her 70s made beautiful jewelry, so beautiful that Saks Fifth Avenue once bought her collection for a mother's day promotion.

Facing challenges with poise

Although she was generally healthy most of her life, Barbara was diagnosed with breast cancer and had both breasts removed in her

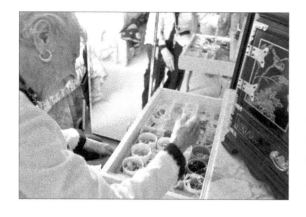

Barbara showing the wonderful beads she used for her jewelry creations.

70s. According to her family, she never complained, never wanting to burden her family. After the operation, she went on with her busy life and the cancer never touched her life again.

Barbara describes her mantra as, "I try not to make a big fuss over things. I always said this too shall pass."

About 10 years ago, Barbara and Arthur moved from Florida to the Classic Residence, a beautiful retirement community in New York. They had a wonderful social life there as they did in Florida. Unfortunately, just a few years later, Arthur passed away from Parkinson's Disease; he was 98. They had been happily married for nearly 70 years.

Barbara continues to stay busy attending various lectures ranging from world affairs to art, teaching residents how to play bridge, creating beaded jewelry (some of which she proudly flaunted during our interview) and remarkably, until she was 101, still practiced Tai Chi.

I would say that Barbara Brody herself is a masterpiece.

REACHING 100 & BEYOND! 102 YEARS

Lifestyle

General health	Barbara is on no medication, "I just take Ensure." Had breast cancer in her 70s and had a double mastectomy. No health issues before or since her surgery.

Smoking	Never smoked ("due to my singing").
Alcohol	Occasionally and moderately.
Nutrition	Barbara cooked occasionally, but her housekeeper cooked most of the time. She ate a variety of foods: meat, salads, blintzes, vegetables, desserts, but never overate. She always ate moderate portions. Per her daughter, "she always knew when to stop and took small portions of her food."
Physical activity	Barbara said that she was never sedentary although she had no rigid fitness regimen. She was never overweight.
Current interests	Attends various lectures from world affairs to art and classes at her retirement residence including exercise, knitting and beading
Family	2 children, her daughter and son both live in NY and see and speak with her regularly; 2 grandchildren and 2 great-grandchildren

Family history

	AGE OF DEATH	CAUSE OF DEATH
Mother	late 50s	heart disease
Father	70s	heart disease
Brother	27	thyroid and heart disease

All of [the art], I soon discovered, were created from Ms. Brody's deft hands and mind's eye.

Nanny, Housekeeper, Minister

Born: February 16, 1911, in Jamaica, West Indies

Current residence: Bronx, New York

WINIFRED THOMAS

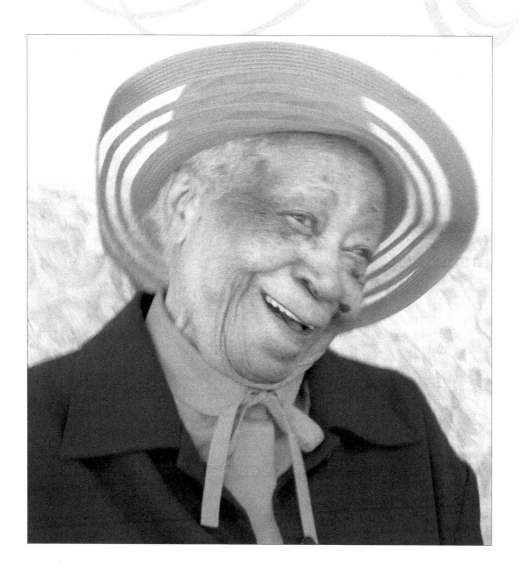

Words of Wisdom

101

*"When you live for God,
talk to him, go to church,
have nice people around you;
that is the best medicine.
God provides for you.
Sometimes you don't know
when it is coming, but it
is coming."*

Winifred Thomas is a very special lady. Her presence and spirit reminds me of another, better known spiritual minister, the great Dr. Maya Angelou. Winifred has a strong, comforting disposition that embraces you like a warm blanket. She is so joyful and passionate about her faith you become captivated by her every word. I barely noticed that she was blind.

A woman of faith and strength

Born in Jamaica, Winifred came to America as a young woman with her mother and settled in New York. She worked in domestic care for a while and went back to Jamaica to raise her family. She gave birth to 8 children, two of whom died as young children.

When Winifred came back to America, she continued her work

"God provides for people in times of need. I witnessed God's work whenever the poor people in Jamaica miraculously found food to survive. God will lead you in every goodness."

She was always there for her children and was a very good seamstress.

taking care of children for other families. She took care of one family for 35 years until she retired. These children adored her so much that they still visit her regularly, even attending her 100th birthday party last year; they were all grandparents by then.

Besides being blind for the past 10 years, Winifred had suffered through incredible loss. She lost 4 of her children, one as an infant, one at 4 years old and the other two relatively young as well, and her beloved husband (to whom she had been wed for more than 50 years) died nearly 25 years ago. "My grandfather, however, lived to be 104," exclaims Winifred.

When I asked her what kept her strong in the face of these challenges, Winifred started to weep. "God provides for people in times of need. I witnessed God's work whenever the poor people in Jamaica miraculously found food to survive. God will lead you in every goodness."

Many people are attracted to "Ms. Winnie's" spirit. Her daughter Cynthia describes her as "outgoing, kind and loving. She was always there for her children and was a very good seamstress. She would sew our dresses and our school uniforms so we didn't have to buy them. She also was a talented pianist and played since she was a kid."

According to Winifred, people would constantly come to her for advice, which she joyfully shared. One strong recommendation of Ms. Winnie's is, "Sow good seeds for your children. Teach your children to give."

Winnie is also a dream maker. One of her grandsons, Dwight, credits his grandmother for inspiring his dream to become a restaurateur. When all of his friends would be playing outside during the holidays, Grandma Winnie would call him inside to help with the cooking, particularly for the holidays. Although he wasn't too happy about missing out on the fun as a child, Dwight learned to love cooking and became very skilled at it because of his beloved grandmother. Dwight says this skill came in handy, especially when he was single and living on his own. His dream is to open an upscale Jamaican restaurant in the near future.

"Sow good seeds for your children. Teach your children to give."

What to do when you are lonely?

Winifred's advice to elderly people who have lost their spouse and are lonely: "Take your Bible and read it, put your burden to the Lord and just leave it there and God will help you."

Besides regularly reading the Bible, Winifred, until recently visited her local senior center four times per week to take dancing and sewing classes.

Lifestyle

General health	Winifred has been healthy her entire life and is on no medication except for eye drops for her blindness.
Smoking	Occasionally for years but quit over 20 years ago.
Alcohol	Occasionally.
Nutrition	Winifred was never overweight and mostly cooked for herself and family. She ate a variety of foods, was not a "big meat or starch eater" and loved vegetables. She also ate very moderately. Some of her favorite dishes were kingfish and red snapper.
Physical activity	Was always active and exercised until recently.
Current interests	Until very recently, she went to the senior daycare center four times per week, participating in dance and sewing classes.
Family	Winifred has four daughters remaining, eleven grandchildren, 24 great-grandchildren and 8 great-great-grandchildren and has visits with many of them regularly.

Family history

	AGE OF DEATH	CAUSE OF DEATH
Grandfather	104	natural causes
Mother	75	unknown
Father	unknown	unknown
Brother	90s	natural causes
Son	infant	unknown
Son	3	unknown
Son	55	unknown
Son	70s	heart disease

Winifred has a strong,
comforting disposition that
embraces you like a warm blanket.

School Secretary, WAC Soldier

Born: October 4, 1915, in Chattanooga, Tennessee

Current residence: Yonkers, New York

SANDRA HOROWITZ

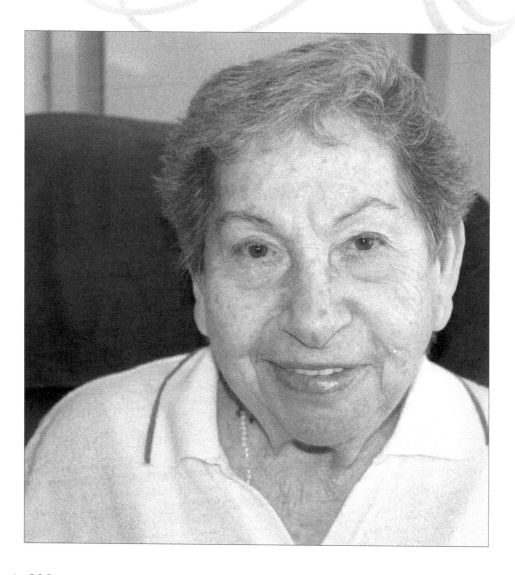

Words of Wisdom

97

*"Keep yourself alert,
active and educated.
Beat to your own drum."*

Sandra Horowitz has not quite reached official centenarian status, but at 97, she is so incredibly youthful, both physically and mentally, she had to be included in our group of inspiring seniors. Sandra lives completely independently at the Classic Residence, a beautiful retirement community in New York. She has no assistance, is sharp as a tack and, most atypical for someone her age, her hearing is perfect.

A woman who wished to save the world

When she was just six years old, Sandra Horowitz moved from Chattanooga, Tennessee to Passaic, New Jersey, as her mother's illness required a different climate. Sandra arrived with a heavy Southern accent. "The kids all made fun of me so I worked very hard to lose it. I did, and now I regret it!" This feeling of regret was not surprising coming from Sandra, a woman who beats to her own drum and is not one to simply conform.

Her strong resolve was even more apparent when Sandra decided to voluntarily serve her country during the Second World War.

It was after the war started, when Sandra and her husband were courting that he felt the need to enlist in the Army. After they got engaged, Sandra, not concerned in the least that she would be one of the first women to serve in the US Army, said, "Why not?" and signed on too.

Sandra became one of the first women to serve with the Army who was not a nurse. She enlisted in the Women's Army Auxiliary Corps (WAAC), which became the Women's Army Corps (WAC) in 1943.

When the WAAC was formed, many men violently opposed it, reportedly fearing that if women became soldiers their own masculinity would be diminished. Other men feared that the women would take all of the non-combat or "safe" positions. Some even went as far as warning their female friends and family that if they became soldiers they would be seen as lesbians or prostitutes.

150,000 women served in the WAC during WWII and they were

> Sandra decided to voluntarily serve her country during the Second World War and became one of the first women to serve with the Army who was not a nurse.

> "Myself and my family all wanted to save the world. However, it was knocked out of me pretty fast. My husband thought I was crazy and was dying for me to get out."

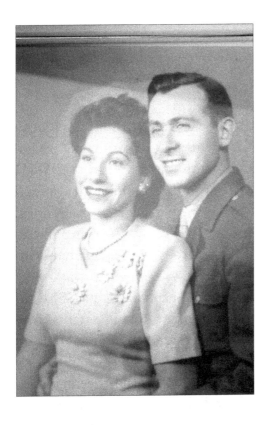

considered by generals, such as MacArthur and Eisenhower, as "their best soldiers." General Eisenhower made this statement: "Their contributions in efficiency, skill, spirit and determination are immeasurable." Although the War Department had considered drafting women at the time, they were too afraid of the public outcry and Congressional opposition, so they shelved the idea.

Racial discrimination rampant in the U.S. Army

Sandra was posted first in Florida and later in Massachusetts. "Myself and my family all wanted to save the world. However, it was knocked out of me pretty fast." She described that when she was serving in KD (kitchen duty) in Massachusetts, she noticed the

> "The women she served with would make lurid racial comments about the black soldiers that were intolerable."

blatant discrimination against the blacks. In her area, the blacks were not allowed out in the field, they all had to serve on garbage duty (unlike how the black soldiers were portrayed in the WWII movies). The women she served with would also make lurid racial comments about the black soldiers that were intolerable to Sandra.

Although he too was serving in the Army, Sandra recalls, "my husband (fiancé at the time) thought I was crazy and was dying for me to get out." She did leave, but not due to his insistence. The WAC began to mandate their soldiers go overseas. Sandra was more than willing to oblige until her mother became seriously ill and she needed to take care of her as most of her siblings had already been drafted.

> "The three of us [Sandra and her children] were in college together!"

Soon after she left the military, Sandra and her fiancé finally wed. Sandra, already 29, was considered "an old maid" in those days and starting to have children in her 30s was almost unheard of. They had two children that she raised with her mother for a few years while her husband finished his call of duty.

Starting a new chapter at 50

While her children were in college, Sandra, at 50 years of age, decided to join them and applied to colleges as well. "I loved school and never had the opportunity to go to college." At a time when so few women barely had a high school degree, Sandra graduated Queens College one year after her older child and one year before her second child's graduation. "The three of us were in college together!"

After graduation, she became a school secretary for 12 years and retired at 68 years old.

"When people say to me 'if you've seen one church, you've seen them all,' I want to hit them! They are all so beautiful and unique with different stories behind."

And at 70

Not one to sit idle, Sandra traveled around the world a few times over as her husband worked for Pan Am Airways at the time. She joyfully described what she and her husband found fascinating and unique about the many different countries they visited including Australia three times, China, Pompeii and New Zealand. Sandra truly appreciates the beauty in art and architecture. "When people say to me, 'If you've seen one church, you've seen them all,' I want to hit them! They are all so beautiful and unique with different stories behind."

Another example of marching to the beat of her own drum is, rather than retiring to Florida like many of her friends, Sandra and her husband moved to Las Vegas for 18 years as they loved the entertainment. They met some very good friends and even took courses at the University in Nevada to nourish their thirst for learning.

After 60 years of a wonderful marriage, her husband died 8 years ago after suffering from an autoimmune disease for 14 years. Following his death, she moved back to New York to an active retirement community.

"What controlled my age more than anything was my mental capacity. I loved school, was always very active at bicycling, tennis and swimming. I like people, always had friends and loved to go to the theatre."

Currently, Sandra, an avid reader, is a member of a library club (once a month), goes to the casino to play video poker on a regular basis, plays canasta weekly and gets involved with the various programs at her retirement community. "What controlled my age more than anything was my mental capacity. I loved school, was always very active at bicycling, tennis and swimming. I like people, always had friends and loved to go to the theatre."

REACHING FOR 100 & BEYOND! 97 YEARS

Lifestyle

General health	Sandra was never seriously ill until she was 89 when she had to have blood transfusions due to a reason unknown. She recovered and has been healthy ever since.
Smoking	Yes, but she quit 40 years ago.
Alcohol	Never.
Nutrition	She was very overweight for a year in her teens while she had pleurisy "while everyone took care of me and fed me constantly." She was very active, quickly lost 50 lbs. and never gained it back. She maintained a good weight, and as she got older had a few extra pounds. She loves fish and chicken with salad and some cooked vegetables. "We always had soup, fruit and dessert with every meal and ate out only once a week. I've never been crazy about meat, but I made veal burgers occasionally. I started taking vitamins at 85 years old, Citracal and Vitamin D."

Physical activity	Avid bike rider, tennis player and swimmer until she was in her 70s. She broke her hips when she was in her 90s.
Current interests	Sandra is a member of a library club (once a month), goes to the casino to play video poker on a regular basis, plays canasta weekly and gets involved with the various programs at her retirement community. She also loves going to the theatre with her daughter.
Family	One daughter who lives out of state but she speaks with regularly, and one son who she sees weekly. She has 3 grandchildren and 1 great-grandchild.

Family history

	AGE OF DEATH	CAUSE OF DEATH
Mother	93	natural causes
Father	52	throat cancer
Brother	n/a	living, age 85
Brother	early 70s	leukemia
Brother	early 70s	heart disease
Sister	62	heart attack

Sandra is so incredibly youthful, both physically and mentally.

HOW HAVE THEY LIVED SO LONG, AND SO WELL?

The people featured in this book were selected not solely based on their extreme longevity; but for their remarkable vitality in their 80s, 90s and even beyond 100. Living a long life doesn't necessarily mean living a quality life. These individuals reached this advanced age with health, purpose and vibrancy. They are helping to redefine aging in new and inspirational ways.

This book is not just about reaching 100. Face it, the majority of us will not. It's about aging with grace and dignity, with purpose and joy—engaging in new social networks, endeavors and adventures that we have never considered before.

Let us explore what these extraordinary individuals had in common and see if perhaps we can incorporate some of their wisdom and lifestyle habits into our own lives.

A mixed bag of genetics in their family

The majority of these centenarians had disease running through their family and managed to avoid it.

Based on the family history noted in each chapter:

- 30% of the centenarians had a parent who lived to 90+ years
- 40% of the centenarians had a sibling who lived to 90+ years
- 80% of the centenarians who had siblings had at least one who died in their 60s or younger from disease, and many of

them had more than one sibling who died much younger, also from disease.

The most relevant statistics to explore are those concerning the siblings as they represent family members of the same generation who grew up under the same conditions and life expectancy, unlike their parents' generation who had a life expectancy that was significantly less. Although 40% of the subjects had a sibling with good longevity, most of the centenarians had at least one sibling who died much younger from disease.

This indicates that we are indeed not doomed by our genetics, nor will they save us. Recent studies reaffirm this notion. According to a new field of genetic research called epigenetics, even when individuals are predisposed to certain diseases in their family tree, they indeed have the opportunity to turn their genetic markers on and off depending on lifestyle factors and mental attitude.

Sense of purpose and humanity

All of these centenarians have made a significant difference in one or more of the following: their family's lives, their community, the world. They all had a strong sense of purpose and humanity, many expressing through their words or actions the importance of helping others.

Some have helped to shape this past century in America and were pioneers in their fields. Dr. Denmark, for example, co-invented the whooping cough vaccine, Ms. Halliday helped change the opportunities in real estate for women, Ms. Gruber saved thousands of Jews from persecution, Ms. Horowitz became one of the first women to serve in the Army, Mr. Ball was part of the first group of golfers to play in the Masters, and Mr. Goldfaden one of the first in the NBA. These just name a few.

Others selflessly and graciously took care of ailing loved ones for many, many years; parents, spouses, even children with Multiple Sclerosis and mental illnesses—and still never complained, even refused help from others. Many of them still participate in some kind of volunteer work.

A compelling collection of recent scientific research has shown that people who volunteer have greater longevity, higher functional ability, lower rates of depression and less incidence of heart disease. Volunteering has been shown to be particularly beneficial to the health of older adults and those serving 100 hours annually, or about 2 hours per week, due to the sense of accomplishment an individual gains from these activities.

Thomas H. Sander, executive director of the Saguaro Seminar at Harvard University, said it best: "Civic engagement and volunteering is the new hybrid health club for the 21st century that's free to join. It miraculously improves both your health and the community's through the work performed and the social ties built."

Basically, it does you good to be good to others! It can greatly improve the quantity and quality of your years.

Generally healthy most of their lives

Ninety-three percent of the centenarians featured in this book avoided all of the serious illnesses including cancer, heart disease, diabetes and Alzheimer's. The few that did contract disease, had it later in life and overcame it rather quickly. None had suffered long, gradual declines in health, physically or mentally.

This indicates that avoiding major illness during your earlier years may allow for a longer life span in general, or perhaps those that have lived the longest have a type of "longevity gene" in their body to help ward off disease. As seen in Mr. Kahn's chapter, the Longevity Genes Project has studied this theory extensively and they have found common genes amongst some "Super Agers", including Irving Kahn and his siblings. Based on this research, Dr. Barzilai, who led the study, is already working on the development of new drug therapies. Very promising, indeed!

Excellent mental attitude and ability to adapt

Each of these centenarians had a sense of humor, was optimistic, and had an ability to adapt to hardship and change. Even with the numerous challenges they faced and tremendous loss they experienced simply due to their advanced age, none were fearful or bemoaned life's difficulties. The most common mantra was, "I go with the tide."

They were all gracious and sociable, exuding warmth, yet independent and strong-willed. It was actually comforting to be in their presence. They were also young at heart. At times I felt as if I were speaking with a contemporary, not someone at least twice my age.

With the exception of the super centenarians (110+), their cognitive abilities and memory, for the most part, were astonishingly intact. They were captivating storytellers, recounting times from as early as 3 years old.

Moderate, balanced food intake = no obesity

New research by the Center of Disease Control and Prevention has shown that obesity is now the leading cause of preventable death in America, causing more fatal disease than the former leader, smoking.

Perhaps our centenarians had this foresight, as none of them were ever obese. A few were somewhat overweight (10 to 30 lbs.) a portion of their lives, but either lost the weight or maintained it, and did not let it get out of their control.

Ironically, only a few of the centenarians were actually cognizant about their dietary intake, but they all said that they just didn't overeat. None of them were vegans, heavy vitamin pill poppers or focused on eating organic food. However, for most of their lives, particularly in their earlier years, they did eat moderate portions of home-cooked, natural foods. Vegetables and fruit were staples on their plates, and meat and starch were eaten in moderate portions, as this was simply the culture at the time. Meat and starch portions then were typically one-half to one-quarter of the size as they are now and vegetable portions and choices were significantly larger and better. Today in America, the leading vegetables consumed are tomatoes in the form of ketchup and pizza sauce, and potatoes in the form of French fries.

Based on my experience counseling many obese clients about their diets, most of their poor eating habits were formed in their early years. These centenarians fortunately molded excellent habits in their formative years. For example, our two oldest super centenarians (114 and 116 years) grew up on a farm eating fresh picked produce and moderate portions of pasture-raised meat.

Unfortunately, our culture of consumption is dramatically

different than the way it was in the first half of the last century, which is why we have the alarming obesity problem in this country. However, it is never too late to incorporate the simple eating habits of our longest-lived people who:

- Consumed mostly foods in their natural form that are ALIVE, meaning those foods that are not heavily processed and will eventually perish if not eaten. This includes vegetables, fruits, legumes, very moderate portions of naturally-raised lean meats with no preservatives, hormones or antibiotics. These "ingredients" were not added to meat in the centenarians' formative years before factory farms were first developed in the 1920s, and not even for years after to the extent that they are incorporated in our food today. Additionally, in those days, a serving of meat was typically 3 ounces, or the size of a deck of cards, unlike the 8- to 16-ounce portions today.

- Consumed moderate portions of grains or starches. In those days, starch portions including pasta and rice were typically no larger than your fist. Today, people typically consume 2 to 4 times that amount at home or in their local restaurant. Refined grains in their day were also not chemically altered like they are today. Since WWII, a laundry list of preservatives have been added to increase shelf-life and to make the product appear whiter.

  Besides moderating your starch intake as did our subjects, it is also very beneficial to switch your grains to ones that are 100% whole. In other words, strive to avoid the "white carbs" (those that say "enriched wheat flour" on the package) and opt for high fiber, less processed and more nutritious grains such as barley, oats, quinoa (pronounced keen-wah), brown rice, whole grain pasta and kasha. They will fill you up faster, keep you satiated longer and improve your digestion; all helpful in reaching your optimal weight and vitality.

- Consumed, if at all, very small amounts of sugar. In America today, the average person consumes 22.2 teaspoons of sugar per day! And the growing intake of sugar over the years goes right alongside with the increasing obesity rate. For many years, health experts have considered sugar to be the most dangerous food you can eat. Excessive consumption leads to a myriad of problems with your insulin leading to diabetes, heart disease, depression, obesity and a host of other illnesses.

    READ YOUR LABELS. Keep in mind that only 4 grams of sugar equals one teaspoon. One 16 oz bottle of Snapple, which typically equals two servings, not one, contains up to 12 teaspoons of sugar alone. Think about how many actual teaspoons, if any, you would add to your tea or coffee. Per the American Heart Association, the recommended sugar intake for adult women is 5 teaspoons (20 grams) of sugar per day, for adult men, it's 9 teaspoons (36 grams) daily, and for children, it's 3 teaspoons (12 grams) a day.

Physically active most of their lives

Not one of these long-lived people exercised as we know it. They didn't frequent the gym, but all have been moderately to very active throughout their lives. About 30% of them played sports regularly for a good portion of their lives (tennis, golf, swimming, dancing, basketball) but all of them were active. Whether it was walking to the store, to work, around their neighborhood or the beach, taking the stairs, tending their gardens or farms, or doing their own yard or housework, they were far from sedentary—their lifestyles involved doing what are referred to as 'NEAT activities.'

Non-exercise activity thermogenesis (NEAT) is a term meaning the energy that is expended for everything we humans do that is not sleeping, eating or sports. Even these minor activities mentioned above have been proven to substantially increase metabolic rate and the cumulative impact of these activities can be a critical component in maintaining body weight.

Therefore, for those of us who dislike formal exercise enough to refrain from doing it, incorporating daily, consistent NEAT activities into your lives will serve to keep up your metabolic rate, which will burn calories and help you reach or maintain your optimal weight.

Remained engaged in mental or physical activity

All of these individuals stayed mentally or physically engaged in activities into their 90s and 100s even if they lost their sight, hearing or ability to walk. Some centenarians were still working as lawyers, financial advisors, real estate CEOs, barbers, lecturers, writers. Most are still involved in volunteer work. Some do the following:

- write books or poems,
- exercise alone or in classes (at local senior centers),
- golf,
- sing or dance (at local ballrooms and in local plays),
- knit,
- travel,
- go to the racetrack,
- read,
- listen to music,
- play piano or the ukulele,
- go to parties,
- make jewelry,
- garden,

- visit family and friends,
- go to church or synagogue,
- attend shows and
- participate in book clubs.

Some even still:

- do their own laundry,
- clean their house,
- cook their own meals,
- drive,
- do their own taxes and
- one even cuts his own hair.

Keeping busy was of vital importance to our interviewees.

Remained connected to their community/family

Many of the activities listed above enabled these centenarians to stay connected and increased their social networks —whether it was with their communities, friends, colleagues or families. They have said that their activities and connections helped keep their minds keen and active. It also staves off feelings of isolation and loneliness.

Never smoked or quit in their early years

Only two of these vibrant centenarians have picked up a cigarette in the past 20 years (one of them still has an occasional cigarette), 63% have never smoked and the rest of them tried it but quit in their earlier years, mostly in their teens to 30s. There were a few who quit in their 50s. One of these centenarians smoked for 30 years and fortunately decided to quit. Two of her siblings continued to smoke and both died of lung cancer, one at 64, the other at 74.

According to the chief medical officer at the American Lung Association, your lungs begin to heal themselves only days after you quit smoking. Inflammation of the airways decreases, breathing starts to become easier and lung function begins to increase. Even exercise capacity improves in just weeks to a few months after cessation. However, if you have been smoking for a long time and have developed COPD (chronic obstructive pulmonary disease—most commonly emphysema and chronic bronchitis), your lungs are beyond total repair.

Regarding lung cancer, the ALA calculates that the smoker's risk can actually return to that of a non-smoker about 10 to 15 years after smoking cessation. However, this depends on the number of years smoking. According to the ALA, the greater the pack years, the greater the risk. When you are getting up around 50 years of smoking and beyond, that's a lot. If people have a lot of pack-years, the risk of lung cancer never goes back down to the risk of a non-smoker.

It is never too late to quit smoking. Quitting will always decrease your disease risk somewhat; but the longer you wait, the more likely you are to significantly decrease your quality of life and even worse, develop cancer. Of course, there are always exceptions to the rule. It seems that everyone knows one relative or acquaintance who had lived to a grand old age while smoking their entire life. They managed to beat the odds. However, smoking causes 87% of lung cancer deaths; thus, the odds are well against you.

Moderate or no alcohol intake

All but two of our centenarians either never touched alcohol or had only an occasional drink, primarily wine, on special occasions or on the weekends. Interestingly, the two who drank more moderately, drank every day, were both male, and both had one to two shots of Scotch!

There is growing epidemiological evidence indicating that moderate alcohol consumption actually reduced mortality among middle-aged and older adults versus abstainers and heavy drinkers. The risk of mortality for heavy drinkers increased 70% due to disease, falls and car accidents. Shockingly, abstainers had double the risk. However, there are other confounding factors that may have affected these results, such as former heavy drinkers who have since abstained and other socio-economic factors. In many of the conclusions, researchers attributed the benefits of the moderate drinking to increased social interaction that has been found to contribute to longevity.

What can you glean from the above information? It will certainly not hurt you to have an occasional drink, or drink reasonably if you choose to, particularly if you are in the company of loved ones and are enjoying your life.

The bottom line

The bottom line is that we all have a chance. A chance of living a long, healthy life filled with purpose and joy. It is just a matter of finding it, not fearing what's ahead. Look at the many activities, ventures and adventures these seniors took on in their platinum years even after facing numerous challenges over their long lives.

They didn't bemoan life's difficulties or think for one minute about how their genetics might affect them. For the most part, they led a clean life, everything in moderation. They "went with the tide," adapted to change and took life on. They stayed on purpose, stayed connected with others and gave generously of themselves.

I hope these humble, remarkable people had the same impact on you that they had on me. I am so blessed for having met them and will keep their wonderful spirits and words of wisdom with me always.

I wish all of you a long, happy and vibrant life!

— Gwen Weiss-Numeroff

ABOUT THE AUTHOR

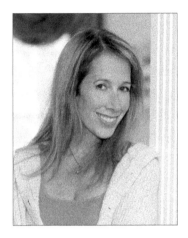

GWEN WEISS-NUMEROFF

Gwen Weiss-Numeroff is a former advertising executive turned nutritionist, professional speaker, and lifestyle coach. In 2001, she founded Corporate Wellness of Hudson & Bergen to help companies keep their employees healthy and productive. She also counsels individuals in her private practice in Pomona, NY.

Gwen made her career switch after witnessing too many loved ones succumb to disease and depression far too early in life. Her mother's sudden death at 70 inspired Gwen to launch a two-year quest to find the secrets to vibrant longevity from those centenarians actually living the dream.

Gwen lives in New City, NY, with husband Bruce and daughters Alexandra and Jaclyn.